Praise for *The Healthy Smoker*

"This is a much needed, comprehensive book about how and why to quit smoking. If you thought you knew it all, had tried it all, but are looking for a way to make it happen (this time!), this is the book for you.

It turns out that you need to prepare to quit smoking, and if you do, you have less trouble quitting! Dr. Bens has a wealth of information on every aspect of getting healthier, supporting your body's wish to be well, and the benefits of specific nutritional supplements. This is information that is specific to smoking, and has never been compiled in just this way before.

Kudos, Dr. Bens, you've filled an important niche. I will definitely recommend this book to my patients who still smoke— that is if they admit it!

—Carol L. Roberts, M.D. Medical Director and Founder Wellness Works, Radio talk show host, WMNF and WHNZ

"The genius of *The Healthy Smoker* is that it is a motivational resource for the smoker AND the non-smoker alike. It's a clear, concise reference guide for those who are truly serious about good health. This is an incredible, must have, book that should be kept with all other timeless references."

—Kathy H. Cramptom, MBA, Director, Convenient Care Centers, Central Dupage Hospital

"The definitive book to quit smoking, and yet this is more than just a book about how to quit smoking, it's a new way of looking at yourself. The wealth of information found in this book is normally found in ten different books, but *The Healthy Smoker* has it all. If you have a friend who smokes this is the perfect gift — it will show you really care. It's also a great book for employers to include in their wellness/prevention program. When you get towards the end and you read about the long-term benefits you'll wonder why you ever did smoke. This book is a must for everyone, even if you don't smoke."

"*The Healthy Smoker* delivers a truly novel way to overcome one of the most common and powerful addictions today. Not only does Dr. Bens enlighten the smoker with many health opportunities, he also eloquently portrays the gradual downfall of a smoking habit. Combined, it offers every smoker a compelling reason to quit, as well as a logical and achievable cessation strategy. A must read to succeed."

"Destined to become a classic, the provocative perspective of this well-written book is engaging and inspiring. Charles Bens brilliantly describes his newly termed 'healthy smoker,' giving comprehensive and intelligent advice for quitting and bringing new meaning to 'better health naturally' for everyone, not just smokers. His refreshing book offers a concise, easy-to-succeed approach that supports one's desire to survive, in spite of less than perfect habits. *The Healthy Smoker* is a major breakthrough and it will not only improve the quality of your life, it may actually add many years which might have been lost."

"Dr. Bens's book has provided renewed hope for all smokers. This book is a seasoned approach to overcoming the smoking addiction based upon proven methods and techniques. Indeed, *The Healthy Smoker* is replete with vital information about good health, health habits, and a smoke-free future.

The Healthy Smoker

How to Quit Smoking by
Becoming Healthier First

Charles K. Bens, Ph.D.

HAPPY CELLS, INC.
Sarasota, Florida

The nutritional and health information presented in this book is based on clinical research and the published experience of various health practitioners, and is true and complete to the best of the author's knowledge. The information provided is not intended to replace or countermand the advice given to anyone by his/her physician. Because each person and each situation is unique, readers are urged to check with a qualified health professional before using any treatment or product where there is any question as to its appropriateness.

HAPPY CELLS, INC.
1327 Cottonwood Trail
Sarasota, FL 34232
Toll free: (800) 737-9617
Fax: (941) 377-7328
E-mail: ckbens@ij.net
www.TheHealthySmoker.net

Library of Congress Cataloging-in-Publication Data available upon request

ISBN 0-9692286-7-8

First Edition

Illustrations and design by Carol Tornatore

Formatting by Susan Zirpoli
Proofreading by Patricia Rockwood

Printed in the United States of America

Contents

Foreword

IMET DR. CHARLES BENS through a mutual doctor friend in Sarasota, Florida. My friend felt Dr. Bens and I had a lot in common in terms of our respect and appreciation for natural medicine. He was right. From the first meeting with Dr. Bens, it was as if we have been life-long friends.

Dr. Bens is easy going, has a great sense of humor and possesses a keen intellect. He is curious by nature, and exhibits a thirst for knowledge, like no other individual I have ever met. I have been involved in several areas of medicine over the past 20 years and have not encountered anyone with such vision, dedication and intense desire to educate and help others.

In terms of Dr. Bens' smoking book, perhaps Mark Twain said it best when he reportedly stated, "I have no problem quitting. I've done it hundreds of times." Since we know that smoking is the leading preventable cause of death in the U.S. and that second-hand smoke takes its toll on non-smokers including children, an alternative therapy, that really works to end nicotine addiction, is desperately needed.

When Dr. Bens first introduced me to the concept of "The Healthy Smoker," it initially seemed like an oxymoron. However, as I examined his research, I began to understand and appreciate the program and its long-term benefits. Smokers who have failed other smoking cessation programs can now follow this simple step-by-step well-designed program and, by first becoming healthy, improve their chances for success.

Thanks to Dr. Bens' dedication and efforts, you, a loved one or a friend has an opportunity to eliminate a terrible addiction and improve overall health and well-being. This book will soon become the "Gold Standard" for anyone motivated to stop smoking by becoming "Healthier First."

—*Stan Headley M.D., N.D., Chief Medical Officer*
of Vaxa International

Introduction

FOR AS LONG AS I CAN REMEMBER smokers have been told they must stop smoking before they can even begin to address any other health issues they may have, such as their need for exercise or their nutritional deficiencies. The reasoning behind this advice was obviously based on the fact that smoking was their biggest health concern; therefore, it should be the thing they tackled first. It occurs to me that this is the very reason why it should not be the first issue or challenge that a smoker should address. Smoking is so big in terms of its addictive grip on the smoker, as well as the daily needs and dependencies it supports, that it would actually be foolish in some cases to tackle it first. It's too big. It's too difficult. And the fact that 70% of would-be quitters fail within three months should be adequate proof of this premise.

In other areas involving addictions there is an accepted practice of gradual withdrawal. The sensible and successful weight loss programs all advise overweight people to lose their pounds gradually in order to be realistic and give the body a chance to adjust. The same is true for heroin addicts or most other changes in personal health. Slower is often better, and there is mounting evidence that this may be true for many people who would like to quit smoking.

There is no question that the cessation of smoking is the best possible goal for every smoker, but does that mean they are doomed to be forever unhealthy because they can't seem to quit? Is it actually possible for smokers to concentrate on other aspects of their health and become healthier in spite of their inability to shake their smoking habit? Haven't we all heard smokers say how healthy their grandmother was even though she smoked for over 70 years and died at the ripe old age of 91? Of course we have all heard this rationalization, and we all know it was just because grandma had good genes, wasn't it? Did anyone ever stop to ask grandma how much stress she had, what she ate, how much physical work she did, or whether she took cod liver oil when no one was looking? If we had stopped to ask, we probably would have learned that grandma had a lot more than good genes going for her.

> **There is every reason to believe that the average smoker could probably be just as healthy, or even healthier, than the average nonsmoker in America today.**

So the question we might ask is, *Can any smoker be healthy just like grandma?* There is no perfect answer that can be applied equally to every person, but generally the answer is probably yes. If you have decent genes and do a lot of things to improve your overall health, there is every reason to believe that the average smoker could probably be just as healthy, or even healthier than the average nonsmoker in America today. That may not be saying much, because the average person is overweight (over 63% of the population), eats the wrong foods, doesn't exercise enough, and is totally stressed out. How hard is it to be healthier than that?

The answers regarding what to do to be a healthier smoker and how to do it are contained in this book. You will have heard some of this advice before, but perhaps not with the same techniques that are aimed at the smoker's perspective and not with the same hope for such encouraging results. When you understand how the body works, and the impact smoking has on the various internal systems, then you will appreciate how the suggestions contained in this book can help you to neutralize or even reverse some of the negative consequences smoking can have on your health.

This book is organized in an easy-to-read and easy-to-follow format with very specific suggestions at each step of the way. If you are able to take action in some or all of the health improvement categories, you will become healthier. Will this book help you to totally avoid cancer or heart disease? No health protocol or procedure can guarantee that, but the advice contained in this book has as much scientific evidence behind it as you will find anywhere for any other health topic.

If you are successful in following the advice in this book there may be a pleasant surprise waiting for you. You may find out that you have actually reduced your body's dependency on nicotine and put yourself in a position for finally being successful in your cessation efforts. I certainly hope so and wish you well in your journey to become a healthy smoker and eventually a healthy nonsmoker.

I. Can Smokers Really Be Healthy?

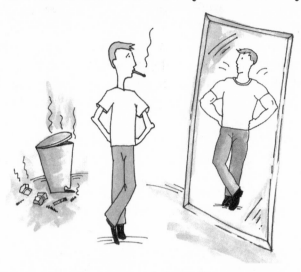

THE NOTION THAT SMOKERS CAN BE "HEALTHY" at first appears as if it is the most outrageous oxymoron imaginable. Many health authorities would say it's impossible for smokers to be healthy because this is the number one health problem in our country causing hundreds of thousands of deaths each year from heart disease, cancer, and many other illnesses. Therefore, conventional wisdom almost forces us to see someone smoking and think to ourselves, there goes an unhealthy person. This kind of thinking is fine as far as it goes, but what if we stop and think about it for a minute. Do you know someone who smokes who actually seems to be healthy? What about the smokers who often justify their terrible habit by saying their grandmother or grandfather smoked and lived to the ripe old age of 91? If even a few of these stories are true, how did this happen? Was it just good genes or good luck that allowed those people to dodge the lung cancer or the heart disease bullet, or could it have been something else?

Healthy Smokers I Have Known
Both of my parents were smokers; one lived to the age of 73, while the other nearly made it to 80. Those ages were about the average

life expectancy for a man and woman born early in the 20th century. Actually, they lived a few years beyond the life expectancy for their generation, and both of them smoked like chimneys for most of their adult lives. In the last 10 years of my father's life he did cut back to four cigarettes per day as well as switching to decaffeinated coffee and only one beer per day. In other words, he used self-discipline to cut back on all of his so-called vices. At the same time he exercised every day by going for long walks and using small hand weights for his upper body. He worked in the garden a lot, ate lots of salad and homegrown vegetables and no junk food whatsoever. He even sprinkled wheat germ on his bran flakes in the morning because he had read somewhere that it was good for you. Remember, he was doing all of this back in the 1950s and 1960s way before the health craze had caught on. He did have one problem: he had been ill as a child and had high blood pressure. He trusted his doctors, who continually tried new drugs on him when the old ones weren't working as well as they should. He worried about this and became somewhat stressed as a result. Certainly, the behavior of his children added to his stressful condition. In my opinion, when he died at the age of 73 he was the picture of perfect health and should have had another 20 years had it not been for his stress and the improper medication from his doctors. Did smoking contribute to his demise? I don't think so. He never had any problems with his breathing, and everything in his medical exams was normal except for that stress and blood pressure problem, which in my opinion was related to many nonsmoking factors.

My mother stopped smoking "cold turkey" at about the age of 70 and lived almost 10 more years until she died of a brain tumor at the age of 79. Did smoking contribute to her brain tumor? Yes, I would probably say that it did, and she became very sedentary in her later years, having worked hard and eaten well most of her life. She had pretty good genes in her family, but nothing extraordinary. She had a chronic cough until she quit smoking, and then it went away, and she was virtually cough and phlegm free for the last 10 years of her life.

Beyond the experience of my parents, I have known many other people who smoked and were, for all intents and purposes, very healthy. I knew athletes who smoked and was constantly impressed by how they could perform even though they would light up right after their event. Over the past several years I did some work for a local ballet company and was amazed to learn that practically every ballerina smoked, supposedly to calm their nerves and help keep their weight down. While these reasons may have been valid in their minds, what was even more incredible was the fact that they could jump around on stage for two hours and never appear to be struggling to breathe. How did they do that, I thought? Some of these young people weren't even eating very well, and they still seemed to be able to endure training and rehearsal sessions that would last seven or eight hours.

The answer to this question of how these and other people managed to look and act healthy started to become clearer at a recent health fair conducted by one of my corporate wellness clients. These fairs are held by employers to help employees find ways to become healthier by getting them to take certain tests and pick up literature on illness prevention. As part of my booth, I invited a company that had just developed a new technology for measuring the level of antioxidants in a person's body. As a reminder, antioxidants are the vitamins and minerals that help support our immune system by neutralizing the free radicals in our bodies. Free radicals are caused by pollution, saturated fat, chemicals in food, and of course smoking. The antioxidants, or the good guys, are vitamin E, vitamin C, selenium, beta-carotene, and zinc, to mention a few. This new technology is capable of measuring the level of these antioxidants at the cellular level by using a special laser light. The employees at this health fair were keen to find out their antioxidant level and lined up by our booth to patiently wait their turn. The highest score possible on this company's antioxidant index is 80,000, and the average is around 19,000 for all people tested so far. A healthy level starts at about 30,000, and the highest person tested at any site is usually about 40,000. I tested at 40,000, but I would have been disappointed if I hadn't tested high given the amount of money I spend on supplements and organic food. The big surprise for me, and for the fellow conducting the tests, came late in the health fair when a middle-aged woman tested at 38,000 and proceeded to tell us that she smoked half a pack of cigarettes every day. How could this be? This has nothing to do with good genes. This is very simply a test of how well our bodies are able to assimilate antioxidants at the cellular level. It was important for me to find out more about how this woman was able to score twice as high as the average fellow employee, most of whom did not smoke. This person ate lots of fruits and vegetables and virtually no junk food. She seemed to have an excellent digestive system with no symptoms of stomach or bowel gas, no constipation, and she consumed small meals throughout the day. She went for long walks every day, had a positive attitude, and took vitamins and minerals regularly. She can't remember being sick and had cut back on her smoking, but had not quit because she still enjoyed a cigarette at certain times of the day. This was not only a "healthy smoker," this was a healthy person. She scored better than all of her fellow employees on our antioxidant test as well as all of the other tests available that day. This was even more impressive since she was approaching the age of 60 while the average age of her fellow employees was about 35. This smoker was healthier than all of the other nonsmokers in her group. Was it because she was doing so many other things that were right? Or was this just some kind of abnormal fluke of nature?

Studies on Smokers
Over the past 50 years there have been many studies on the impact of smoking as it relates to a person's health. These studies never produce statistics indicating that 100% of smokers will get lung cancer or 100% of smokers will get heart disease. There is always a certain percentage of any test group, such as 20, 30 or 40%, who seem to escape the ravages of this unfortunate habit. There is hardly ever any explanation offered as to why some people do get lung cancer and others don't. Recently, there have been some studies that have indicated that the people without lung cancer seem to have

more vitamin A (beta-carotene) in their bodies. Another recent study found that smokers who take vitamin C (at least 900 mg/day) are 70% less likely to have a stroke than smokers who do not take vitamin C. A Scandinavian study found that smokers taking beta-carotene actually were more susceptible to heart attack than smokers who were not taking beta-carotene (a synthetic form of beta-carotene was used). How can this be? This discrepancy in the findings of various studies often stems from the medical community's insistence that only one vitamin, drug, or condition be tested at a time. Unfortunately, this is not how the human body works. Vitamins and minerals work synergistically to help one another do their respective jobs within our bodies. Vitamin E supports vitamin C, selenium supports vitamin E, and so it goes that vitamins and minerals need each other in order to be effective. This is not the case with prescription drugs, which usually work independently of one another and thus can more accurately be tested in these "so-called" single variable studies.

> Vitamins and minerals work synergistically to help one another do their respective jobs within our bodies.

The same phenomenon occurs when tests are done on smokers. It is almost always simply a test of smokers versus nonsmokers with very few other factors taken into consideration. Sometimes age grouping is done, and sometimes specific employee groups are selected such as the famous Framingham Nurses Study on diet and heart disease. Very rarely are people asked how much they exercise, how many supplements they consume, or how many vegetables they eat. It would appear from the previous examples that these factors indeed should be taken into consideration, because this may be the reason why some smokers become ill while others do not. The study previously mentioned, where smokers taking vitamin C had a 70% less probability of having a stroke, certainly begins to point in this direction. What if all of the people not becoming ill from smoking not only had good genes but also were doing other things to improve or protect their health like eating right, exercising, taking supplements or practicing yoga? What if a study was done on the three million people who quit smoking each year and it was found that many of them had adopted some of these other healthy habits which actually made it easier for them to quit? No one has looked at this possibility, but given the evidence, albeit small at this point, that smokers can maintain a fairly high level of health, maybe this theory needs further study.

What if the smokers who became the most ill were also the people who were the most overweight, who exercised the least, who took the fewest vitamins, and who ate the most junk food? What if it were those factors, as much or even more than smoking, that made them ill? Once again we bump up against the very unscientific tendency of testing just one factor instead of a number of them. Could it be that multiple negative factors can make you ill, and multiple positive factors can help to keep you healthy? It makes common sense and yet we are just starting to get into the testing of multiple factors. This type of testing may be more difficult to do, but given the questionable accuracy of the single variable studies it appears to be time to move away from them if we are to get more scientifically valid study results.

Smokers Must Quit First
Since smoking is always put at the top of the list of lifestyle health risks, conventional medical wisdom has always been that smokers must quit smoking before they can do anything else about improving their health. Smokers who really don't want to quit have had a built-in excuse for not exercising, not eating better, or not taking supplements because those things presumably won't do any good until they stop smoking. The aforementioned evidence seems to be indicating that this might not be true, and some smokers seem to have already figured this out.

> Maybe, just maybe, it would be better for most smokers to take a different approach and try to become healthier before they try to quit.

Maybe smokers don't need to quit in order to begin to become healthier. Maybe they can even become healthier than the average nonsmoker, because the average nonsmoker is not eating right, is overweight, doesn't exercise, and doesn't take supplements. Over 63% of the population is overweight. According to the Centers for Disease Control only 1% of the population get all of the nutrients they need every day. About 60% of the population take some form of supplements, but many are taking very cheap supplements which probably aren't absorbed very well by the body. And, while 60% of the population say they get some form of exercise every week, there is some doubt that they are exercising seriously.

And so it would seem that smokers could actually become as healthy, or even healthier, than the average person with the adoption of some relatively easy lifestyle changes. They don't need to quit first. In fact, it would probably be easier and smarter for some people if they didn't try to quit first. Smoking is a terribly strong addiction, stronger than heroin or cocaine addiction according to some scientists and medical doctors. Maybe, just maybe, it would be better for most smokers to take a different approach and try to become healthier before they try to quit.

II. The Strength of Smoking's Addiction

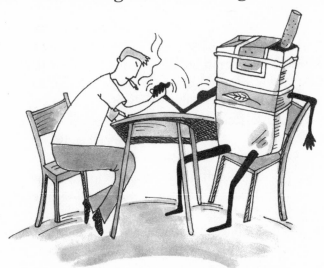

E VERY SMOKER WHO HAS TRIED TO QUIT "THEIR HABIT" knows exactly how addictive smoking is. Obviously, some people have a more difficult time than others because some people manage to quit cold turkey the first time they try, while others fail over and over again. There have been numerous studies trying to identify why this happens, and the best that science can come up with is:

- Some people are genetically more prone to addiction than others.
- Some people have more willpower than others.
- Some people have stronger physiological needs than others.

Our purpose here is not to reinvent all of these studies in the search for a definitive answer on the reasons for addiction. Rather, we would like to look at smoking in terms of the relative difficulty of quitting compared to other desirable lifestyle changes.

Smoking is one of the strongest addictions known to mankind, even stronger than smoking crack cocaine or injecting heroin, according to many scientists and doctors. The Surgeon General of the United States says that smoking is more costly and deadly on a national scale than heroin, cocaine, and alcohol. Further evidence on the strength of tobacco addiction can be seen in the percentage of people who are successful in their efforts to quit. An average of 70% of smokers who try to quit are smoking again within three months. And 90% of smokers would like to quit, have tried many times, but just can't seem to get the job done.

In spite of the extreme difficulty involved in kicking "the habit," doctors and health officials continue to tell people that they must quit if they ever hope to be healthy again. As we have seen in the previous chapter, this may be less than helpful advice for some people who find it difficult to quit smoking but may not find it as difficult to adopt some other lifestyle changes that can improve their health. Some people have found their way to better health by changing other things in their lives other than their "smoking habit," and that's what we would like to explore now. What are these other lifestyle or health changes, and exactly how easy or difficult are they to do compared to the cessation of smoking?

> An average of 70% of smokers who try to quit are smoking again within three months.

We have selected 17 lifestyle or health improvements in order to show the relative difficulty involved in making such changes. These are arbitrary selections, and this is not a scientifically determined measurement of difficulty. It is based on a review of the scientific literature and then an extra portion of comparative difficulty based on my assessment. In other words, this is my best guess at the relative difficulty of each lifestyle or health change based on the many books I have read. These relative difficulty comparisons are shown in Chart I using five levels of difficulty from not very difficult to change to extremely difficult to change. Smoking is the most difficult change, and taking supplements or using natural therapies are among the easiest things to change.

The first four items on the chart are the addictions experienced by many people around the world and include smoking, taking drugs, alcohol consumption, and caffeine use. The other 13 items are all

CHART I
HEALTH CHANGE DIFFICULTY

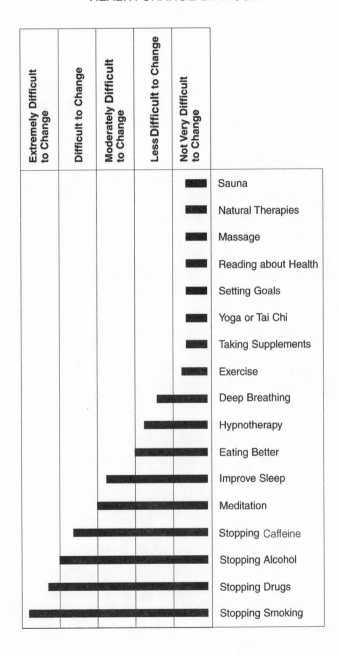

Extremely Difficult to Change	Difficult to Change	Moderately Difficult to Change	Less Difficult to Change	Not Very Difficult to Change	
				▬	Sauna
				▬	Natural Therapies
				▬	Massage
				▬	Reading about Health
				▬	Setting Goals
				▬	Yoga or Tai Chi
				▬	Taking Supplements
				▬	Exercise
			▬▬		Deep Breathing
			▬▬▬		Hypnotherapy
		▬▬▬▬			Eating Better
		▬▬▬▬▬			Improve Sleep
	▬▬▬▬▬▬				Meditation
	▬▬▬▬▬▬▬				Stopping Caffeine
▬▬▬▬▬▬▬▬					Stopping Alcohol
▬▬▬▬▬▬▬▬					Stopping Drugs
▬▬▬▬▬▬▬▬▬					Stopping Smoking

lifestyle or health changes that have been adopted by many people to improve their health. Of course, it must be stated that stopping any or all of these addictive behaviors would also have a very significant impact on the improvement of a person's health. The difference is they, the four addictive items, are much more difficult to change precisely because they are addictive. The other 13 items are not addictive by comparison, although some doctors will tell you that exercising can become addictive due to the "adrenaline rush" many people experience after exercising.

Our hypothesis is based on this question: What if a person adopted several of the health improvement items instead of, or at least before, he or she tried to quit smoking? Could they become healthier? Would it make it easier for them to quit smoking? Let's take a brief look at some of the health-promoting categories.

Reducing Stress
Most smokers will tell you that smoking calms their nerves and gets them through the tough parts of the day, even though science tells us the reverse is really true. Smoking has some calming effects, mostly psychological, but eventually increases stress through the increased release of adrenaline and cortisol. What if a smoker used other stress-reduction strategies such as deep breathing, meditation, yoga, tai chi, taking B vitamins, and eating calming foods such as vegetables and nuts instead of less calming foods like sugar and caffeine? Such actions might reduce the psychological and the physiological need for tobacco and allow the smoker to cut back on his or her dependency on smoking.

> Smoking has some calming effects, mostly psychological, but eventually increases stress through the increase of adrenaline and cortisol.

Improving Sleep
Many smokers have a difficult time sleeping because their nervous system is on edge and they crave nicotine during the night. What if the smoker took some melatonin, calcium, and magnesium at bedtime to help induce the sleep process?

Taking vitamin B12 in the morning also helps to strengthen the sleep cycle. Calming audiotapes have been successful for many people. Avoiding caffeine, especially after dinner, will help considerably in the ability to secure a good night's sleep. There are several herbs that have a good track record as sleep aids, including catnip, chamomile, lavender, lemon balm, passion flower, and valerian. Some homeopathic remedies also help such as coccalus and gelsemium. If sleep can be improved, a person's overall health will greatly benefit and the smoker is no exception.

Eating Better

Many smokers depend heavily on their cigarettes and coffee (with lots of sugar) to get them through the day. The sugar spikes their glucose and insulin levels, and when they come down from this sugar high they use cigarettes' help to pick them up. By eating a decent breakfast with complex carbohydrates and protein, the body can avoid these peaks and valleys, as well as give the cells something for repair and new cell development. Eating plenty of fruits and vegetables throughout the day will boost the immune system, provide the necessary vitamins, minerals, and enzymes for bodily functions, and bring the body back into balance. The vegetables will also help keep the body in an alkaline state, which will make it very difficult for any disease to grow. These benefits accrue to the smoker as well, especially as he or she consumes fruits and vegetables with high levels of vitamin C. Smoking depletes vitamin C, leaving the body vulnerable with a depressed immune system. By changing a few key eating patterns, a smoker can neutralize many of the negative aspects of smoking. Heart disease and cancer, two of the most common diseases of smokers, can be reduced by 50 to 70% with the consumption of seven to nine helpings of fruits and vegetables every day. (This reduction is for the general population and may be less for smokers.)

> **Heart disease and cancer, two of the most common diseases of smokers, can be reduced by 50 to 70% with the consumption of seven to nine helpings of fruits and vegetables every day.**

Taking Supplements

Everyone agrees that we should all get as many nutrients as we can from the food we eat. It is also common knowledge that it is impossible to get all of our necessary nutrients from food due to the depletion of our soil, transportation and storage time, the use of pesticides, the processing of food, and the cooking of food. The loss of nutrients due to these depleting aspects ranges from 20 to 80% depending on the type of food and the severity of the depletion events. Therefore, everyone needs supplements, especially smokers. A good multiple vitamin would be a minimal approach along with extra amounts of vitamins A and C. Vitamin A is especially useful for the lungs, and vitamin C is the best antioxidant for smokers. Of course, vitamin E is a helper to vitamin C, and selenium is a helper to vitamin E, so they would also be wise choices. There are a few other nutrients that the body has difficulty getting from the food we eat, and they include essential fatty acids (omega-3 especially) and minerals such as zinc, calcium, magnesium, and potassium. Specific amounts of these supplements are not mentioned here because everyone's need is different. Suffice it to say that the RDA (Recommended Daily Allowance) is much too low, and it would be wise to consult a nutritionist or a doctor trained in nutrition. By providing the body with the nutrients it needs, anyone, including smokers, can become healthier, thus avoiding minor illnesses such as colds and flu as well as the more serious diseases such as diabetes, heart disease, stroke, and cancer.

> By providing the body with the nutrients it needs, anyone, including smokers, can become healthier.

Exercising

Many smokers don't exercise because they say they get out of breath too easily. Still others use smoking as an excuse not to exercise because they say they will start their exercise program just as soon as they stop smoking. This is a classic "Catch 22" situation, because many people never quit smoking so they never start exercising. Well, your excuse is now officially taken away. Many smokers have been able to simply start walking a little every day

16

until they increased their breathing ability to the point where they could walk at a brisk pace for 30 minutes or longer. This is all it takes to get a tremendous benefit in terms of the reduced risk of disease. Improved circulation will help to reduce the risk of stroke and heart disease as well as assist in delivering nutrients to the cells and removing waste material from them. Metabolism and digestion should be improved, which will provide additional help with detoxification and the uptake of nutrients. If some resistance exercise can be added in, all the better for muscle tone, burning of calories, and increasing bone strength. Exercising as just described is not that difficult to start or to maintain, especially when it is compared to the difficulty of stopping smoking.

Reading About Health
Knowledge is power, and the more you read about how to become healthier the more you will be motivated to do so. Even reading an article or two each week will make a difference, because the information will start to accumulate and create a subconscious argument for the necessary changes in your lifestyle. Going to a newsstand to pick out a magazine on health is painless, and the benefits can be tremendous. Additional years of healthy living and the avoidance of pain and suffering are priceless benefits. Remember these are not substitutes to stopping your smoking habit. These are strategies you can easily do in order to become healthier so you can eventually quit. What is easier than reading? If you are reading this book then you have already taken a big step forward, but there is much more to learn, and this knowledge is literally at your fingertips in articles, books, or online.

Setting Goals
Everybody sets goals, but most people don't keep them. Why? Probably because they were too difficult in the first place. This is precisely why this book was written. The goals a smoker can set for himself or herself have just become incredibly easier to reach because they are not nearly as difficult as the cessation of smoking. You don't need to do all of the health improvements mentioned in this chapter all at once. Pick a few of the ones you think you would

really like to start with and get them well established in your daily routine. Then gradually add another and another until you start to feel healthier. Once this happens you will be amazed at how reluctant you are to go back to being the old you. You may even be amazed at how much less dependent you are on smoking and how much easier it is to quit.

Natural Remedies

There is an entire chapter on natural remedies for smokers, such as acupuncture, yoga, and meditation, just to mention a few. In fact, one of these natural remedies may be the place where you want to start your journey to better health. Read them over and pick the one you have always wanted to try. Every one of them has been proven to be effective as a means of both preventing and, in some cases, helping to remedy various health challenges.

III. Smoking's Impact on Your Body

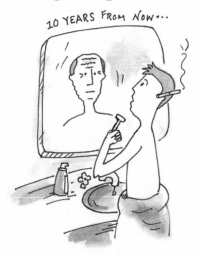

M OST SMOKERS HAVE HEARD ABOUT ALL OF THE BAD THINGS that happen to your body as a result of smoking, like cancer, heart disease, and wrinkled skin, so why go over this again? The reason is simple and important. Unless you know all the exact impacts of smoking, you may not be as ready as you should be to take the necessary counter-measures this book is recommending. When you fully understand how each vitamin protects your body, even if you smoke, then you will be much more likely to remember to take that vitamin pill. The same is true for all of the natural therapies and treatments recommended. So please, read this chapter carefully and keep this information in mind to help motivate yourself to adopt the various lifestyle changes recommended.

> Unless you know all the exact impacts of smoking, you may not be as ready as you should be to take the necessary countermeasures this book is recommending.

The Physiology of Smoking
There are four distinct phases of change that the body experiences during the process of smoking. By understanding these physiolog-

ical changes a smoker can better appreciate the importance of the various Healthy Smoker strategies.

Phase One – Inhaling tobacco smoke causes nicotine to enter the bloodstream and go immediately to the brain. Once in the brain nicotine stimulates the release of serotonin and dopamine neurotransmitters, which provide the "good feelings" of relaxation or even excitement. The receptor cells in the brain that receive these neurotransmitters soon become less sensitive to this stimulation. This requires higher and higher doses of nicotine to produce the same level of stimulation.

Phase Two – Very shortly after nicotine reaches the brain it also reaches the liver, which triggers the release of sugar into the bloodstream. The added sugar produces a feeling of energy for the smoker, which, combined with the feel-good sensation in the brain, gives the smoker an overall feeling of energy and concentration. These sensations are very temporary because they are chemically stimulated rather than being produced by nutrients that are more sustainable.

Phase Three – Due to the release of sugar into the bloodstream the pancreas reacts to release insulin needed to help deliver sugar to the cells as well as keep sugar levels balanced in the body. Sugar levels are temporary and excess insulin results, since the pancreas thought real food was the cause of the increased sugar levels. This causes sugar levels to drop lower than they were before the cigarette. At the same time neurotransmitter release also stops because it was also short term. This combination of stalled neurotransmitter release and low blood sugar produces feelings of fatigue, irritability, hunger, and craving for another cigarette. This cycle usually takes about 15 minutes.

Phase Four – As blood sugar and neurotransmitter levels are falling nicotine stimulates the nervous system to release adrenaline into the body. This causes increased heart rate and respiration as well as a feeling of tension which, combined with the feelings of fatigue and craving, causes the desire for another cigarette. This is precisely how the body reaches a state of addiction.

This cycle interrupts regular eating patterns which, in turn, causes the body to experience imbalances due to nutritional deficiencies. Chemicals take up residence in the cells as antioxidants lose their ability to neutralize the excessive free radicals being consumed. The cells, in an effort to protect themselves, surround themselves with cholesterol causing the cell membrane to become harder and less subtle. This restricts the ability of cells to take in nutrients and excrete waste products, which weakens cells. The cells begin to age prematurely and become vulnerable to illness and disease.

Primary Impacts of Smoking
The chart on the next page graphically depicts all of the ways that smoking can impact your body. These impacts occur gradually over a long period of time, and every smoker may not experience all of them. However, there is enough clinical evidence to suggest that many smokers will experience many of these conditions after 20 years or more of smoking and sometimes sooner. The reasons for these impacts are generally attributed to the introduction of free radicals in the smoke that is inhaled, the increased stickiness of the blood, and the reduced bioavailability of nutrients needed for cell growth and repair. Each impact has some specific characteristics that deserve attention in order to properly appreciate the value of making changes in certain aspects of your life.

Stress – Nicotine causes your body to produce more stress hormones such as adrenaline and cortisol, more thromboxane, and less prostacyclin. These changes cause your heart rate and blood pressure to increase. When your body is under stress on a very regular basis, this weakens your immune system, making you vulnerable to illness.

Stroke – Nicotine, stress, and the tar in many cigarettes causes your arteries to constrict. If the blood vessels in your brain constrict, this can restrict the amount of oxygen getting to the brain, resulting in a stroke.

Brain Tumor (cancer) – Smoking releases many free radicals into your body that can damage cells when they try to replace their missing electron with one stolen from one of your cells. If this happens in the brain, a tumor can begin and grow over many years if the body's immune system is weak and unable to neutralize these free radicals.

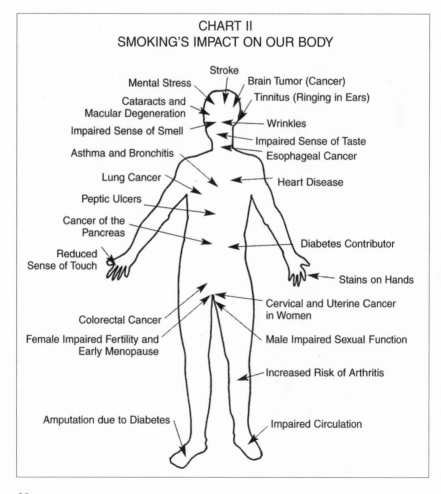

CHART II
SMOKING'S IMPACT ON OUR BODY

Stroke
Mental Stress
Brain Tumor (Cancer)
Cataracts and Macular Degeneration
Tinnitus (Ringing in Ears)
Impaired Sense of Smell
Wrinkles
Asthma and Bronchitis
Impaired Sense of Taste
Esophageal Cancer
Lung Cancer
Heart Disease
Peptic Ulcers
Cancer of the Pancreas
Reduced Sense of Touch
Diabetes Contributor
Stains on Hands
Cervical and Uterine Cancer in Women
Colorectal Cancer
Female Impaired Fertility and Early Menopause
Male Impaired Sexual Function
Increased Risk of Arthritis
Amputation due to Diabetes
Impaired Circulation

Tinnitus – Ringing in the ears can be caused by the inability of the inner ear to get the nutrients it needs or remove toxic materials. Smoking can contribute to this because of the narrowness of the blood vessels involved and the stickiness of the blood, the coating of cholesterol and plaque used to repair damaged blood vessels.

Cataracts and Macular Degeneration – The eyes are just as vulnerable as the ears when it comes to tiny blood vessels that can become blocked. Smoke also dries the exterior of the eyes, adding to the degeneration process. Nutrients are not able to reach the eyes to keep them functioning as they should. Without adequate levels of certain carotinoid vitamins the eyes begin to deteriorate, and this can eventually lead to the creation of cataracts.

Wrinkles – Smoking causes wrinkles in at least two important ways. The first is the constriction of blood vessels caused by nicotine. The second is the impact smoking has on the destruction of vitamin C. Every cigarette destroys at least 25 mg of vitamin C, which is responsible for the production of collagen, which in turn is responsible for holding our connective tissues together.

> Every cigarette destroys at least 25 mg of vitamin C, which is responsible for the production of collagen, which in turn is responsible for holding our connective tissues together.

Taste, Touch, and Smell – Nicotine decreases each of these senses through its toxic effect as well as the decreased circulation to our nerve endings.

Mouth and Esophageal Cancer – Smoking irritates the mouth and the throat. It also causes the cells of your mouth, larynx, and esophagus to be attacked by the free radical toxins present in tobacco smoke. This can lead to serious irritations, which can then lead to the production of cancerous cells.

Asthma and Bronchitis – When the lungs are irritated and nicotine paralyzes the cilia, excess mucus remains in your lungs where it can create a perfect environment for bacteria and viruses. Many smokers wake up during the night to cough up the mucus being stored in this way because the cilia become unparalyzed at night when they are not being subjected to nicotine. However, with only a brief seven or eight hours of relief, this is not enough to negate the damage done during the day, which leads to problems such as asthma and bronchitis.

Lung Cancer – This is one of the biggest problems for smokers, since smoking involves the inhalation of carbon monoxide, acetone, formaldehyde, vinyl chloride, hydrogen cyanide, hydrogen sulfide, and many other toxic chemicals. These gases cause the overproduction of mucus in our lungs, the paralysis of the lung's natural cleansing mechanism, and the weakening of the immune system's ability to respond to viruses and bacteria. This creates the perfect environment for the development of cancer.

Peptic Ulcers – Many of the chemicals in cigarettes irritate the lining of the throat as well as the stomach. These irritations can lead to ulcers as the stomach's lining is compromised. Stress caused by cigarettes adds to this problem.

Heart Disease – Heart disease is the second most prevalent negative impact of smoking. The chemicals in tobacco produce free radicals, which travel through our arteries destroying cells and causing plaque to be built up. This eventually leads to blockages, which in turn lead to heart attacks. Nicotine can also cause the heart to beat vigorously, which does not help the situation at all. It was also mentioned earlier that smoking causes the blood vessels to constrict, leading to increasing heart rate and blood pressure. This combination of events makes smoking very heart unhealthy.

Colorectal Cancer – Over 4,000 chemicals (toxins) are in each cigarette and many of them are carcinogenic. The carcinogens find their way into the digestive system through the bloodstream and the food we consume, leading to cancer in the colon.

Female Infertility and Early Menopause – Smoking causes a serious disruption to a woman's hormones as well as blood flow to her reproductive organs. This can lead to a decreased production of fertile eggs as well as an early cessation of making them. The result is early menopause, which can trigger other health problems such as vaginal dryness, night sweats, hot flashes, and the increased risk of osteoporosis.

Male Sexual Problems – Nearly two-thirds of impotent men smoke, almost twice the rate of the general population. Decreased circulation to the penis is caused by the same problems causing decreased circulation to other parts of the body such as constriction of blood vessels, the build-up of plaque, and stickiness of the blood. The number of men having poor circulation to their penis is 300% higher in smokers than in nonsmokers.

> The number of men having poor circulation to their penis is 300% higher in smokers than in nonsmokers.

Pancreatic Cancer – Several studies have concluded that people who smoke and drink coffee and/or alcohol have a much higher risk of pancreatic cancer than the average person who does not smoke or drink coffee and/or alcohol. Toxins and poor circulation are the same reasons for pancreatic cancer, which is true of many other cancerous situations related to smoking. Smoking also inhibits the production of vitamin B, which is needed by the pancreas, as well as antioxidants needed to fight free radicals and cancer cells.

Diabetes-Related Problems – Diabetics who smoke are eight times (800%) more likely to have complications than those who do not smoke. Since diabetics also have circulation problems, smoking can make these problems worse, thus leading to the increased likelihood of an amputation being needed for a foot with gangrene.

Arthritis – The drying of the joints is certainly accelerated with smoking, which leads to inflammation and the deterioration of joints.

As stated earlier in this chapter, these health problems often take many years to develop and often are not detected until they are well advanced. The build-up of plaque in the arteries and blood vessels occurs so slowly that we don't even notice it. If our blood pressure does go up due to this build-up, the doctor may simply give you a prescription to lower your blood pressure, which does not address the basic problem.

The same is true for asthma, bronchitis, or a chronic cough, all of which could be due to smoking, but the symptoms are suppressed by prescription drugs. This suppression of symptoms does very little to resolve the underlying problems of the destruction of cells in your throat or your lungs. All it does is give you a false sense of security about your health, which continues to decline in spite of the control of the symptom.

Aging is also blamed for some of the symptoms we begin to experience due to smoking. After all, wrinkles are just another sign of aging as are deterioration in hearing or eyesight. Never mind that these problems are occurring 20, 30, or 40 years before they should be due to smoking. They happen to most people eventually, so we think it was just our turn, and we do what we can to mitigate or control them in some way. We get glasses for our eyes or have an operation of some kind. We use creams for our wrinkles or get a facelift. We take more drugs for our stress and our heart problems so that by the time we are in our sixties the average smoker is already on five to ten prescription medications. If men experience sexual problems they just get Viagra.

And so we spend our lives suppressing all of these messages our body has been trying to send us until it is too late. The body can't compensate forever, and the drugs only deal with the symptoms in most cases. When cancer or a heart attack occurs we may finally realize that we waited too long. Then the medical establishment throws the really big "solutions" at you like bypass surgery,

26

radiation treatments, or chemotherapy. None of these medical "solutions" are pleasant and in many cases they actually hasten death.

If there is any single message to be taken from this chapter, it is the amazing ability of the body to compensate for the harmful things we do to it and the harm we do when we suppress these symptoms that the body sends us. The standard medical tests provided at an annual check-up cannot detect most of the problems created by smoking in the early stages. That means there are only three logical strategies available for the smoker who wants to become healthier:

> The standard medical tests provided at an annual check-up cannot detect most of the problems created by smoking in the early stages.

1. Understand the serious illnesses associated with smoking and take the preventative measures spelled out in this book.
2. Get the tests recommended in this book on a regular basis in order to get better indications of your true health, which are not provided by the usual medical exam.
3. Avoid taking the prescription drugs that suppress your symptoms in favor of more natural approaches that address the root cause of your health problem.

The Cost of Smoking

The impact of smoking goes beyond what happens to the human body. There are serious financial impacts as well. Everyone has seen figures on the overall cost of smoking to our economy, but they are worth repeating because they add valuable incentives for those who are trying to quit as well as the people who employ them. The Centers for Disease Control estimate that 46.2 million people smoke and that they are responsible for $75 billion per year in medical expenses and $80 billion per year in lost productivity. Any company without a stop smoking incentive program is losing plenty of money, and unfortunately, many of the programs that do exist don't work very well. If these companies adopted the Healthy

Smoker Program they might finally be able to get a decent return on their stop smoking program investment.

The individual smoker should be aware that the cost of smoking for them goes well beyond the direct cost of the cigarettes, which averages about $4.00 per pack. Duke University found that the actual cost of a pack of cigarettes for a 24-year-old person is about $40. The factors influencing this dramatic cost include the money lost on the resale of houses and cars, increased insurance cost, teeth cleaning, dry cleaning of clothes, lost work time, and shorter life spans.

A breakdown of these cost factors proves the true financial impact of smoking on an individual. A one-pack-a-day smoker will spend about $1,600 per year on cigarettes alone. A 40-year-old person who quits smoking and puts his or her savings on cigarettes in a 401K at 9% interest would have $250,000 in that account by age 70. The average loss on the trade-in of a car is about $1,000, and a thorough house cleaning and painting could cost over $2,000 if a smoker wanted to get top dollar for his or her house.

Insurance costs are also much higher for smokers. Term life insurance can run about $3,000 per year more for a $500,000 policy, and health insurance is about $200 per year more. Over a lifetime of smoking (50 years), the extra cost for smokers can get up to $200,000, and we haven't even considered homeowner's insurance. Smokers also pay into social security and company pension plans but receive much less in pay-outs because of their shorter life span. Add up all of the breath mints, dry cleaning, dental cleaning, and other "smoker's costs" and it is easy to understand how the $40 per pack cost occurs.

Any smoker should take these costs into consideration when thinking about the advantages of quitting. Providing for one's family and not exposing them to secondhand smoke are strong motivational factors that can help smokers to stay focused on their cessation efforts. Recent reports have revealed that over 80% of the population do not have an adequate savings plan for retirement. Wouldn't it be great if the Healthy Smoker Program could not only make you healthy but secure your retirement as well? Putting $1,600 per year or even more into your 401K could provide a secure retirement for any family.

The cost of smoking is about $200,000 over a lifetime, and the potential investment return of not smoking is about $250,000. The next time you light up, think about the nealry $500,000 (half a million) you are throwing away.

Note: For more on the cost of smoking in the workplace please go to www.ash.org/papers/n100.htn.

IV. Testing the Health of Smokers

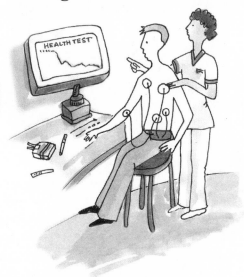

IN AN EARLIER CHAPTER I BRIEFLY DISCUSSED the difficulty of diagnosing many of the long-term health consequences of smoking. Part of this difficulty stems from the smoker's unwillingness to admit there could be a problem developing, and part of it stems from the inadequacy of many existing medical testing procedures. Even if some health problem is diagnosed, there is a strong tendency to treat the symptoms rather than the root cause of the problem. That is why it is so important that smokers not only change their attitudes, but that they also avail themselves of some better, more advanced health diagnostic procedures. The following tests have proven to be extremely effective in the early diagnosis of many of the health challenges which may confront smokers.

Oxygen Test – This test scans the tip of your finger to determine how much oxygen is circulating in your system and reaching your cells. This is vital for smokers since nicotine inhibits the delivery of oxygen by the hemoglobin in our blood. The highest score is 100, but if a score drops to the low 90s, it means that oxygen delivery is being impeded. Further tests may be required to determine the exact reason and what can be done to correct the problem. A naturopath or holistic medical doctor can be of assistance in this situation.

Lung Capacity Test – This is a standard test given to asthma patients to determine how much lung strength or capacity is present. By asking the client to blow into the test unit the health practitioner can measure the volume of air exhaled and inform the client if there has been any loss or gain since the previous test. This test is invaluable for smokers since the lungs are the most threatened part of the body for them. The cilia in the lungs are paralyzed during smoking and thus cannot perform their cleansing action. The subsequent build-up of mucus can inhibit lung function. When smokers start an exercise program, this test can help motivate them as they begin to see improvement in their lung capacity.

Blood Pressure Test – Smoking can have a major impact on blood circulation, which in turn can increase the heart rate and blood pressure. It is important to test blood pressure on a regular basis because it can fluctuate for so many reasons including stress, exertion, eating, etc. Even slight changes, which show a consistent trend, should be examined further to determine the cause.

Heart Disease Test – Although cholesterol has been the test of choice for heart disease for many years, there is mounting evidence that there are other tests that are equally, if not more, important. Getting your blood tested for the presence of C-reactive protein, homocysteine, fibrinogen, and triglycerides is very important, especially for smokers. These tests are not that expensive, are usually covered by insurance, and can provide an excellent early warning to the development of heart disease and/or arteriosclerosis.

Live Blood Cell Test – Most conventional medical doctors will tell you they don't believe in this test, but that is primarily because they don't understand it. This test looks at a sample of your blood under a microscope and can detect irregularities such as sticking platelets, deformed blood cells, blood cells with inadequate hemo-globin, or the presence of yeast and parasites. This information can be invaluable to smokers as an early warning of the damage being done by smoking and provide an opportunity to take important corrective measures.

Stress Test – There are a number of different stress tests including a written survey to identify patterns of stress, or a treadmill test to test heart recovery rate. This is an important area to test for any smoker because smoking gives the temporary feeling of relaxation but also increases the production of stress hormones such as cortisol and adrenaline. Blood tests for these negative hormones would be yet another way to determine if stress is becoming a factor in maintaining good health.

Antioxidant Test – There is a new technology that can determine the level of antioxidants in your body. A safe laser light is used to scan your hand to detect the presence of a broad spectrum of antioxidants in your cells. For smokers this is important to know since smoking destroys antioxidants, thus lowering the body's immune system. Low immune function makes us vulnerable to illnesses of many kinds, and it is possible to rectify this problem with changes in diet and/or supplementation.

Glucose Test – Testing for sugar levels can provide an early warn-ing in the development of diabetes. Smoking not only contributes to the development of this disease, it also causes more severe con-sequences such as amputations due to poor circulation. If upward trends in sugar levels were detected it would be possible to use exercise, dietary changes, supplements, and herbs to bring this condition under control. This would help to avoid the need for prescription drugs as well as prevent diabetes.

Eye Test – Smoking contributes to macular degeneration as well as cataracts and glaucoma, so it makes sense to have your eyes checked on a regular basis. If dryness is starting to occur or eyesight is deteriorating, these may be signs that smoking is having a negative impact on your eyes. There are definitely measures that can be taken to slow down or even reverse this problem, including diet and supplements.

Hair Analysis – You may ask what the hair has to do with smoking? Our hair keeps a very precise record of what is happening in our bodies in terms of the vitamins, minerals, and toxins present. Clippings of undyed and unpermed hair can be analyzed for a very small fee and yet provide a wealth of information. Most naturopaths or holistic medical doctors can arrange for this test and then help develop a strategy to address any nutritional imbalances or toxins that might be found.

Vitamin Analysis – Blood tests can also be used to determine the level of vitamins and minerals in the body, although this will give a more short-term perspective. Hair and body cell tests are better for longer-term analysis. The advantage of blood tests is that they can also include markers for the presence of cancer and other problems, as well as being covered by most insurance plans. Our blood is the ultimate carrier for all diseases and can be an invaluable overall test.

Thermography – Thermography is a relatively new test although forms of it have been around for several years. It uses thermal imaging to detect the level of heat coming from the body. Inflammation, which is an integral sign of nearly all diseases, creates heat levels higher than the body's usual temperature of 98.6 F. This is why thermography is used to detect the presence of cancer cells. Thermography is totally safe and involves no touching of the body, radiation, or pain as is the case with mammography. Diseased organs or tissues can be detected in their early stages and allow for treatment or remedial measures to be taken.

pH Test – It is extremely difficult for disease to be present in a person with an alkaline body. A simple test of urine or saliva in the

> **It is extremely difficult for disease to be present in a person with an alkaline body.**

morning, using a test kit from the drug store, can reveal the acid/alkaline level of the body (7.2 – 7.4 pH [desired range]). If a high acid level exists, this could be a sign for the need to switch to a more alkaline diet (i.e., fruits and vegetables). The value of this test has been scientifically researched and proven, and it can be one of the best early warning signals for future health problems for anyone, including smokers.

Bio Meridian – This is one of the most sophisticated diagnostic tools available in the field of natural health and is sometimes referred to as Electro Dermal Scanning (EDS) or Evaluation According to Vol (EAV). This equipment measures the electrical output of the body's systems and organs, which increases under stress and declines after years of toxicity or nutritional deficiency. Many European doctors use this type of equipment, and some North American practitioners are starting to follow suit. This machine can determine the health of your internal organs well in advance of most tests used by conventional medicine. Most communities now have a Bio Meridian practitioner, and smokers would be well advised to find this person to do periodic analysis of their overall health.

V. Detoxification Before Anything Else

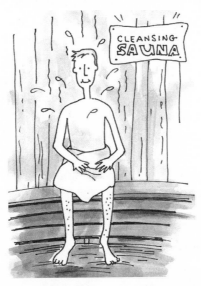

Our bodies are constantly challenged to cope with an onslaught of toxic substances coming from many different sources. Every cell in our body, and there are over 60 trillion of them, is involved in an ongoing detoxification process. If our cells are successful in their detoxification efforts, we can expect to live a long and healthy life. If they are not successful we will experience unnecessary illness and likely die prematurely. If you didn't care about this process and didn't want to learn more about it you wouldn't be reading this book. Knowledge is power, so understanding where these toxins come from, how your body deals with them, and how you can help your body to deal with them better is the focus of this chapter. Even if you quit smoking it would still be extremely helpful to make a special effort to rid your body of the toxic materials that have accumulated over the years.

> If our cells are successful in their detoxification efforts, we can expect to live a long and healthy life.

Where do toxins come from? There are many outside sources of toxins as well as harmful events that produce toxic reactions in the body. The following list will give you some idea of the range and seriousness of these sources.

Smoking – Thousands of toxic chemicals enter your body every time you smoke, making this one of the most toxic conditions a human body can experience.

Water – Municipal filtration systems do not remove many of the toxins that seep into our water supplies. Even the chlorine and fluoride that are added to the water are toxic to our bodies. The government's claim that the water from your tap is safe to drink is only partially true. From an immediate perspective, it is usually safe to drink, which means you won't get sick immediately after drinking the water. What they don't tell you is that the long-term implications of drinking tap water can be extremely harmful. The accumulation of toxins in the body over many years of drinking most tap water has been proven to contribute directly to many forms of cancer.

Food – The food we eat is full of pesticides and other toxins leaching into our food through the air and water that plants consume, as well as directly from the soil. If you are a trusting person you tend to believe the claims of the government and agri-business that the food is safe, but several scientific studies have verified the presence of many cancer-causing chemicals in much of the food we consume.

Radiation – We are bombarded with radiation from x-rays, computers, television, airplane travel, and a host of other sources. This radiation produces free radicals in our body and lowers the strength of our immune system.

Air – We are constantly breathing toxic substances from car exhaust, factory emissions, secondhand tobacco smoke, and toxic substances emanating from the earth (e.g., radon). Our body must cope with this chemical stew and get rid of it as quickly as possible. The longer it stays in our body, the more harm it can cause.

Stress – Increased stress causes the brain to encourage the development of harmful hormones such as cortisol. These harmful body chemicals can damage our arteries and cause imbalance in many bodily functions.

Clothes – Even the clothes we wear can contain chemicals. Some clothing contains chemicals in the form of dyes, and dry cleaning also uses very toxic chemicals. These toxins are absorbed through the skin and must be dealt with by the body's detoxification process the same as those toxins that are consumed with water or food.

Teeth Fillings – Mercury is one of the most toxic substances on our planet, and many people still have fillings in their mouths that contain mercury. This mercury can leach into our bloodstream and poison many parts of our body.

Prescription Drugs – Some drugs are vitally important and help people overcome serious health challenges. Unfortunately, drugs are grossly overprescribed and are treated by our body as if they were chemical invaders. Our liver and kidneys are often severely damaged due to the overload of prescription drugs.

> Our liver and kidneys are often severely damaged due to the overload of prescription drugs.

Work Exposure – Many workers are exposed to toxic substances every day, and this has been proven in many successful lawsuits over the years. Health and safety laws are better today than they were many years ago, but millions of employees continue to be exposed to dangerous chemicals on a daily basis.

Household Exposure – Even in our homes we are exposed to toxins in the building materials used to construct our houses, the carpets we walk on, and even the pans we cook with (e.g., Teflon).

The point of presenting this partial list of toxic exposures is not to induce a feeling of terror or doom, but rather to awaken you from the usual complacency and apathy that most people have. If you are aware of these dangers and do nothing about them, then there should be no surprise or remorse if you succumb to them someday in the form of some serious illness or disease. The problem is not knowing which toxin has "done you in." There are so many, and cancer doesn't announce that it has been caused by a particular chemical. We know that certain substances like nicotine or mercury are more toxic than some other substances, but we haven't been able to figure out which combination of toxins actually conspire to cause a particular health problem. Maybe someday we will.

What is a logical detoxification strategy?
Obviously, the first line of defense is to avoid any toxins that you can. Here are some basic strategies:

- Quit smoking or cut down the amount you smoke.
- Drink filtered water or spring water from proven safe sources.
- Eat organic food as much as possible.
- Reduce radiation with fewer x-rays (most aren't necessary) and less time in front of the television or computer.
- Use quality air filters in your house.
- Reduce stress with yoga, deep breathing, more vitamin B, or eliminating stressors.
- Wash new clothes before wearing them.
- Hang drycleaned clothes outside for a few days to allow chemicals to disperse.
- Wear natural fiber clothing (cotton and wool) with minimal chemical treatment.
- Get your mercury fillings replaced.
- Avoid prescription drugs by seeking out safer herbal remedies.
- Urge your employer to have an independent analysis done to detect workplace toxins.
- Have your house tested for the presence of toxins, including fungus, and take corrective measures when necessary.

These are good ideas for avoiding future exposure to toxins, but what about the ones that have already accumulated in your body? Anyone who doesn't think they have toxins in their body is naïve and in danger of courting some disease in the near future. Here are some of the symptoms that indicate you have toxins in your body.

• Allergies or odor sensitivities
• Headaches or nasal congestion
• Bad breath or a coating on your tongue
• Body odor
• Respiratory problems
• Brittle nails or dry hair
• Insomnia
• Depression
• Chronic fatigue
• Unexplained weight gain
• Constipation
• Skin problems

> In some cases, the liver can be damaged by as much as 70% before any signs of liver disease will show up in standard medical tests.

These are just some of the more noticeable symptoms of toxicity in the body. Even if some of them are not yet present, this does not mean that you are not in a toxic state. The body is truly amazing in its ability to adjust and compensate for our foolish behavior. In some cases, the liver can be damaged by as much as 70% before any signs of liver disease will show up in standard medical tests. Kidney stones can grow in size and number before any pain or discomfort occurs. Cancer can advance to impact several feet of your colon before any pain or signs are experienced. If you wait until you have symptoms, you have already waited too long.

Attacking Toxins Logically
If you already have some toxic symptoms, or even if you don't, there is a logical plan of attack for detoxification because toxins accumulate in certain parts of your body. That is not to say that

toxins can't be everywhere in your body, because they can. However, there are established toxic pathways and cleansing centers in your body where cleansing efforts should be concentrated.

The liver is the body's primary detoxification center performing the following amazing functions.

- It manufactures 13,000 different body chemicals.
- It maintains 2,000 internal enzyme systems.
- It filters 100 gallons of blood on a daily basis.
- It produces one quart of bile daily.

Why does the liver produce or process all these materials?

- The bile is used for the digestion of fat.
- The liver makes and breaks down hormones including cholesterol, testosterone, and estrogen.
- The liver controls the regulation of blood sugar.
- The liver filters all food, nutrients, drugs, alcohol, and materials in the blood.
- The liver is part of the immune system that alerts the body to the presence of pathogenic microbes and toxins.
- The liver detoxifies all internally or externally produced toxins.

Detoxification Cautions
Detoxification is not suitable for some people and may even be dangerous if certain conditions are present. The following types of people should only use detoxification under the watchful eye of a qualified health practitioner.

- Someone with a terminal or malignant illness.
- Someone with a genetic disease such as an inherited metabolic problem.
- Someone with a mental illness of any kind.
- Someone with an autoimmune disease.
- Someone suffering from hyperthyroidism.

- Someone who takes medications regularly.
- Someone who is pregnant.
- Someone who is chronically underweight.
- Someone who has chronic or acute liver or kidney problems.

Detoxification may likely help many of these conditions, but the risk of some negative reaction strongly suggests the need for appropriate monitoring throughout the detoxification process. A holistic medical doctor or a naturopathic doctor can provide the best advice on the level of detoxification needed as well as the appropriate monitoring program.

If you were only going to detox one part of your body, the liver would be the one to select. There are many good books available to help guide the liver detoxification process, but one of the best is *Renew Your Life* by Brenda Watson. A basic liver detoxification program would include:

- A diet consisting of fruits, vegetables (beets, spinach, carrots, cabbage, and especially cucumbers), fish, chicken, eggs, good oils (flaxseed, olive), good clean water, and fiber.
- Nutrients (supplements) including lecithin, vitamin C, vitamin E, selenium, alpha lipoic acid, NAC (N-aceytl-cysteine), amino acids (especially taurine and methionine), and calcium D-Glucarate, a powerful detoxifier.
- Herbs are also very helpful, including milk thistle, dandelion, green tea, and turmeric.
- Special supplements to consider include DMG (N, N-Dimethyl Glycine), Colloidal Silver, and Newton Homeopathic #1 Detoxifier.
- There are also several good liver detox teas that can be included in a detoxification program.

If you can accomplish a cleansing of your liver following a plan similar to one described above, you can do more to improve your

" . . . cleansing
of your liver . . .
can do more to
improve your
overall health
than almost
anything else
you can do. . ."

overall health than almost anything else you can do with the exception of quitting smoking. And, you should detoxify even when you do quit smoking in order to clean out the residue of many years of toxic behavior. A special liver detoxification supplement has been developed for smokers by Vaxa International. Ordering guidelines can be found in the back of this book. *(See* Appendix I.)

The next obvious place where toxins accumulate, especially for smokers, is in the lungs. There are many great books with programs for cleaning out the lungs, but one of the best is in the book *Prescription for Nutritional Healing* by James Balch, M.D. Some of the suggestions from this and other books include:

- A diet exactly like the one described above for the liver with the addition of soy foods, guavas, pumpkin, watercress, wheat germ oil, raw fruits, raw vegetables, and tomatoes.
- Supplements such as the ones listed for the liver plus beta-carotene, MSM, vitamin B complex, vitamin B12, quercetin, and vitamin A.
- Herbs such as astragalus membranaceus and cordyceps also help.

An excellent supplement to assist in the cleansing of the lungs is available from Vaxa International. Vaxa Lung Formula promotes the body's natural process of respiration while providing nutritional support for the lungs. This formula is a blend of homeopathic remedies, along with herbs rich in key nutrients traditionally known for their value in naturally supporting lung function like lungwort, white horehound, coltsfoot, lung moss, garden violet, and soap bark in a base of minerals and trace elements traditionally used to support lung function. Do not be fooled by the peculiar-sounding names of these ingredients, which were named years ago by Asian and European healers who first identified their very specific healing properties. (Guidelines for ordering the Lung Support formula can be found in Appendix I.)

Obviously, an exercise or deep breathing program will also help in your lung detoxification efforts. Getting clean air in and the bad air out is always good for the lungs. There are other parts of the body that can also benefit from specific detoxification efforts. The lymph glands are the collection and holding areas for toxins before they are sent to the liver for processing. Lymph massage helps to push these toxins out of the lymph glands for better processing. Be careful not to push too many toxins toward the liver because it is possible to overload the liver and create a toxic backload. Always use a qualified lymph massage person for this cleansing technique.

Another key detoxification area is the intestine. There are many different cleansing techniques including hydro-colonic therapy, which is quite a dramatic event the first time it is experienced. The colon is actually flushed to remove all of the encrusted fecal material, which can cause cancer of the bowel as well as other toxin-related diseases. Other less dramatic detoxification efforts include the use of a high fiber diet with foods such as rice, bulgur, figs, parsnips, asparagus, garlic, and brussels sprouts. These foods not only help to cleanse the colon but also help to combat the cancers that attack this part of the body.

Perhaps the easiest and the most effective detoxification strategy is to engage in a total body detoxification program. One of the truly superior detoxification programs available comes from Vaxa International, one of the leading research-based homeopathic medicinal companies in North America. The ingredients in Vaxa's detoxification product have been proven in clinical trials and in practical application for many years by thousands of health practitioners. The program consists of a specially formulated supplement, which is consumed as a pill at specific times of the day. (*See* Appendix II for the list of ingredients.) There is also a special diet to follow, which basically omits dairy products, gluten-containing grains, and citrus fruits. A typical meal is shown in Appendix III. Vaxa International provides a one-month supply of the supplement as well as a diet guide to help insure effective detoxification.

There are other cleansing possibilities for the kidneys, the bladder, and the skin, but perhaps the best overall cleanse for smokers involves the elimination of heavy metals from the body. This can be accomplished most effectively with chelation therapy, which usually involves intravenous treatments that remove heavy metals from the blood. This type of cleansing has been safely and effectively used for over 50 years. Heavy metals such as mercury, aluminum, lead, cadmium, and others are among the most toxic substances entering the body and eventually cause heart disease, cancer, and many other health problems. There are also oral chelation formulas that are very effective. They take a little longer to remove the heavy metals than intravenous chelation but they are less expensive and less time-consuming. The final chelation possibility is the use of suppositories that are also very effective but not preferred by some people.

The skin is the second most important detoxification organ after the liver. The best way to draw toxins out of the body and through the skin is to use a regular sauna, an infra-red sauna, or a steam bath. Be sure to drink plenty of water and follow the advice of a qualified health practitioner.

Common Reactions During Detoxification
Detoxification is a very powerful cleansing process that can produce some strong bodily reactions. These reactions are usually mild but can be more serious in some people. Anyone beginning a detoxification program should be aware of these potential reactions and be ready to take the appropriate measures in response.

1. **Swollen throat** – Usual cause is inflamed lymph glands. The antidote is to drink parsley tea until the swelling subsides.

2. **Dizziness** – Usual cause is low blood sugar. The antidote is increased fluids and rice intake.

3. **Diarrhea** – Usual cause is increased fiber from fruits and vegetables. The antidote is usually eating more rice.

> Detoxification is a very powerful cleansing process that can produce some strong bodily reactions.

4. **Constipation** – Usual cause is lowered food intake. The antidote is to consume rice protein shakes and more ground flaxseeds or flax oil. Additional vitamin C or magnesium may also be helpful.

5. **Flu-like symptoms** – Usual cause is germ and toxin flushing from the sinuses. The antidote is to cut back on detoxification product and plan the beginning or restart of the program for the weekend.

6. **Nausea** – Usual cause is bile stagnation. The antidote is a lemon and water drink with a pinch of cayenne pepper on waking.

7. **Excessive weight loss** – Usual cause is lowered caloric input of people with a fast metabolism. The antidote is to increase protein powder and ground flaxseeds in protein shakes.

8. **Headaches** – Usual cause is dehydration, caffeine withdrawal, or liver congestion. The antidote is increased water intake and perhaps a natural remedy such as lavender. (Usually applied as an aromatherapy oil on the temples or as vapor for breathing.)

9. **Insomnia** – Usual cause is low blood sugar and liver congestion. The antidote is a fruit shake before bed or a homeopathic remedy such as Newtons Detox #1 at bedtime. Melatonin, inositol, or DHEA may also be helpful.

10. **Rash** – Usual cause is body toxin elimiation. The antidote is a cool bath or compresses, a poultice made with chaparral, or an oil such as tea tree.

11. **Intestinal gas** – Usual cause is increased vegetable fiber intake. The antidote is one charcoal tablet after each meal or digestive enzymes before the meal.

12. **Irritability or fatigue** – Usual cause is low caloric intake. The antidote is more rice protein shakes during the day. Add almonds, an apple, and molasses for more serotonin.

These symptoms or reactions during detoxification are quite common and indicate that the program is working in most cases. Using these antidotes and staying with the program is usually the most desirable course of action. However, if these reactions continue or get worse it is probably best to stop the program and consult with your health practitioner about the best course of action to follow.

Conclusion
Some people might say, *"Why bother to detoxify if you are still going to smoke?"* The answer is very simple. If you can rid your body of nearly 90% of the toxins that are in it, would this make you a healthier person? The answer is obviously yes. In three separate studies, smokers who ate raw vegetables, fruit, and green vegetables every day reduced their risk of lung cancer by 59%, 44%, and 52% respectively. There is mounting scientific evidence that smokers can reduce their risk of most diseases if they help detoxify their bodies by eating the right foods, taking the right supplements, and following some other basic detoxification and cleansing programs.

VI. The Digestive System

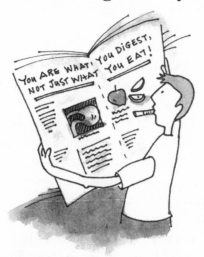

You Are Not Just What You Eat; You Are What You Digest

A FTER A SMOKER HAS CARRIED OUT a detoxification program, it is time to begin thinking about how to optimize the nutrient intake of the body. This is crucial because every cell in the body, all 60 trillion of them, is replaced on a regular basis (with the exception of brain cells). Our outer skin and the lining of our intestines are replaced every two weeks. Some cells, like those in bones and cartilage, are denser and thus can take months to be replaced. As we age, the process takes longer, which means it is even more important to ensure that everything we eat is high quality food full of vitamins, minerals, and amino acids. It is equally important to ensure that all of this nutritious food is actually digested and put to use replacing those old cells and building a strong immune system.

Smoking can have some very negative impacts on this digestive and nutrient intake process. Therefore, any smoker who wants to become healthier had better pay attention to the recommendations for improving digestion. Here are some of the key factors to consider in the improvement of digestion.

The Food Purchased – It all starts with the food that is bought because everyone should know by now that whole natural foods are the best. Our bodies are designed to eat plants, as you can tell by the type of teeth we have. Carnivores, or meat eaters, have ripping and tearing teeth, while we have grinding teeth. Carnivores also have short intestines (six feet usually) so the meat can go through quickly, while our intestines are much longer (approximately 24 feet). This longer intestinal system is custom built for eating plants. Over the years (thousands and thousands of years) humans have become accustomed to eating meat, and now our bodies require some of the key nutrients in meat such as iron, amino acids, and B vitamins. As a result of this adjustment most people need some meat to remain healthy, although fish and fowl are by far the best choices. Red meat is the most difficult food to digest and causes many health problems if eaten in excess. Too much protein consumption can cause calcium to be leached from our bones and flushed from our bodies through urination. Too much meat can also contribute to heart disease and various cancers, especially cancer of the colon.

When we use the terms whole and natural foods, we mean as close to a natural state as possible. Breads and cereals should have whole grains and seeds in them with no refined flour or chemicals of any kind. Fruits and vegetables should be fresh and organic, not canned or frozen. Foods that have not been processed in any way and have been purchased from local growers, if possible, will be the best foods in terms of nutrients and digestion. The longer it takes for foods to get from the ground to your plate the more nutrients and enzymes are lost.

> The longer it takes for foods to get from the ground to your plate, the more nutrients and enzymes are lost.

Any person, and especially smokers, can make a big difference in their overall health by purchasing fresh whole foods. More will be presented later on the ideal diet for smokers. The remainder of this chapter will concentrate on other factors impacting digestion.

The Preparation of Food – Digestion is definitely affected by how food is prepared or cooked. As a general rule, the more you cook food the worse it is in terms of nutrient value lost and impeded digestion. Enzymes are destroyed at high temperatures, which means vegetables should be lightly steamed or eaten raw. Even meat should not be overcooked, although it is important to cook all meats thoroughly enough to kill all bacteria or other harmful organisms. Microwaving is not good for food because it alters the molecular structure of the food thus making it less available for the body to use. Some raw fruits and vegetables should be consumed every day in order to provide the necessary fiber to keep the digestive process working well. Without adequate fiber from whole grains, seeds, raw fruits, and raw vegetables it is easy to become constipated. This blocks the digestive process by not allowing nutrients to be properly absorbed. It also can lead to the excessive production of toxins in the intestine, which can put a strain on the immune system.

Smokers can ill afford to have more toxins coming into their bodies from a constipated or inefficient digestive system. One of the best ways to even partially neutralize the toxins being taken in from smoking is to optimize the nutrients coming into the body. Almost every "healthy smoker" I have encountered has a great digestive system through the purchasing of whole foods and the proper preparation of those foods. This allows them to produce healthy replacement cells as well as give a much-needed boost to their immune system.

The Eating Environment – Believe it or not, it makes a big difference where you eat and the environment you eat in. If you eat in a quiet and relaxed place, this greatly improves the possibility of good digestion. Eating on the run is silly and should be avoided at all costs. Most people think that as long as they get something in their stomach, the body will be able to make something good out of it. That is only partially true. The body can take some energy from almost any food, but if it is consumed in a stressful environment there may be too much stomach acid present or the blood needed for digestion may be somewhere else in the body. Eating slowly and in a familiar quiet place will optimize the digestion of your food.

How You Chew – Chewing is critical because if you don't break the food down completely, it cannot be digested properly. Chewing induces the production of enzymes in your saliva, which starts the digestive process for carbohydrate foods. The digestion of proteins starts in the stomach with different kinds of enzymes, but they can only be effective if the protein is properly chewed. Some nutritionists say we should chew our food 30 or even 40 times before swallowing. Of course, this depends on the type of food you are chewing. The main thing to remember is to ensure that the food is not in chunks but rather totally chewed to a near liquid state.

The patience of chewing is good discipline for smokers who may have a tendency to be in a hurry. This rush may be general habit or even be triggered by the desire to get to the next cigarette sooner. Regardless of the reason, the act of chewing can bring many rewards in the form of patience, reduced stress, enjoyment of the food, and excellent digestion.

How Often To Eat – The frequency of meals and time between them plays an important role in the digestive process, which also impacts the ability of the body to get the highest level of minerals and vitamins from the food we eat. This is especially important for smokers who can ill afford to miss any of the available nutrients in their diet. Most progressive nutritionists agree that it is important to eat five or six small meals every day. At the very least, we should eat three medium-sized meals and a few very healthy snacks in between (one between breakfast and lunch and one between lunch and dinner).

Eating every three hours ensures a steady supply of nutrients to our cells as well as a steady source of energy. Metabolism is also balanced, which helps to keep the body's cleansing process in top operating condition. Smokers need to flush toxins from their bodies as often as possible. Eating one or two bigger meals puts a strain on the digestive process and can impede the regular metabolic processes within the body.

> Eating every three hours ensures a steady supply of nutrients to our cells as well as a steady source of energy.

Obviously, these small meals should all consist of natural foods. The body needs large quantities of complex carbohydrates, vegetables, fruits, healthy oils, and lean meat or vegetable proteins. More specific nutritional guidelines will be provided in the next chapter.

The Sequence of Eating – Why do you think it is a good idea to eat a salad at the beginning of your dinner or a piece of fruit 20 minutes before your lunch? The answer is enzymes. The body needs enzymes in order to properly digest the food we consume. Our bodies make some enzymes but also need the enzymes that are found in raw fruits and vegetables. Heating food destroys or greatly reduces the amount of enzymes in our food, so it is important to eat some raw or very lightly steamed vegetables or fruits at the beginning of each meal, if possible. These enzymes help to break down the food entering our bodies, which helps the assimilation of nutrients. This may seem like a small or inconsequential action, but over many years the increased intake and digestion of nutrients, such as antioxidants, can have a dramatic impact on the ability of the body to neutralize the free radicals we are exposed to. This oxidative process is what causes the body to age as well as become vulnerable to illness and disease. Smokers can ill afford to miss this opportunity to help their bodies absorb higher levels of nutrients through this intake of valuable enzymes.

Hydrochloric Acid and Enzyme Levels – Did you know that hydrochloric acid levels in the stomach and enzyme levels in the body diminish with age? This is part of the natural aging process that gradually reduces the level of nutrients going to our cells, which in turn triggers the slower replacement of those cells. This is what we call aging, but it doesn't need to happen as soon or as quickly as it normally would. Stomach acid (hydrochloric acid) often declines because of an insufficient intake of zinc. Zinc is difficult to get nutritionally, so it may be necessary to use supplements to help ensure the body gets enough (30-40 mg/day). It might also be helpful to use digestive enzyme supplements, which can help the digestive process. There are even some digestive enzymes that contain a small amount of betaine hydrochloride. One of the best products of this type is Nature's Lining by Lane Laboratories. Clinical tests have proven the ability of this product to reestablish a stomach lining and good stomach acid balance within a few weeks.

Your Flora Levels — Even if you have taken all of the previous steps to protect your digestive process, there still has been very little actual digestion of nutrients until food gets into the small intestine. When food arrives in the small intestine there must be plenty of friendly bacteria to accomplish the final breakdown of the food for absorption by the body. Absorption happens through the intestine walls and into the bloodstream. Friendly bacteria, often referred to as acidophilus-bifidus and other similar names, must be present in order to accomplish this transformation of partially digested foods into nutrients. Many people are out of balance in terms of the bacteria in their intestines due to the intake of antibiotics and other prescription medicine. These drugs destroy both friendly and unfriendly bacteria, which then impedes the digestive process and allows for the spread of candida (bad bacteria). This can lead to infections in various parts of the body, such as vaginal infections in women or skin rashes and blood infections in men and women. Foods such as yogurt contain acidophilus, but it is usually necessary to take acidophilus supplements to rebuild the friendly bacteria to satisfactory levels. Smokers cannot afford to miss this very simple and inexpensive solution to this bacteria imbalance. By keeping their friendly bacteria levels high, smokers can ensure good digestion (assuming they have followed the previous guidelines), keep themselves free of candida and fungus infections, and ensure the highest possible nutrient intake.

Metabolism – When people say they have a fast or a slow metabolism what does that mean? Generally, it is considered the rate at which your body breaks down food and makes it available for cell rebuilding and energy as well as how fast toxic material is removed from the body. Smokers need to ensure they have the fastest and most effective metabolism possible on both counts, because they need all of the nutrients they can get and the least amount of toxic material. Smokers already take in more toxins through smoking than they should, so it is incumbent on them to optimize nutrient intake and toxin outflow.

Metabolism is improved by ensuring the sufficient intake of fiber in the form of raw fruits and vegetables, as well as whole grains and seeds. Exercise is also an important factor because body movement helps to encourage the movement of food through our systems. The presence of certain vitamins and minerals also helps metabolism by increasing the conversion of food to energy. The breakdown of glucose in food into energy depends on the presence of vitamins B1, B2, B3, B5, and C, iron, and Co Q10. The actual transport of glucose to the cells depends on the presence of vitamins B3, B6, chromium, and zinc. We don't get these vitamins and minerals from junk food, which means our metabolism becomes sluggish and we put on fat when we eat this type of food. Smokers who are cutting back on their habit, or even quitting, often complain about putting on extra weight. That may be partially due to putting more food into their mouths in place of cigarettes, but it is even more likely to be due to the fact that they are not exercising, not eating nutrient-rich foods, and not consuming enough fiber. If they did all of these things, as well as follow the other guidelines in this chapter, they would probably not have to worry about poor metabolism or weight gain.

Digestion at the Cellular Level – The digestive process is very complex as can be seen by the previous abbreviated explanation. However, if a smoker intends to compensate for his or her smoking habit by trying to eat and digest the healthiest foods, there is one more important step to consider. After food is broken down in the small intestine and goes into the bloodstream as nutrients or is sent to the liver for storage, it still must be delivered to our cells for utilization. We each have about 60 trillion cells, so this is a very busy process that requires speed and efficiency every step of the way. If we have done everything perfectly up to the point of nutrient transport, we still may not get all of the nutrients into our cells if our cells have a hard, and difficult to enter, outer surface (membrane). Nutrients need to pass through the cell wall for proper utilization, and then the waste produced by the cell needs to pass back through the cell wall for transport to the liver and kidneys, where the waste is prepared for exit from the body.

The outer walls of our cells can become hard and difficult to penetrate due to smoking and eating a poor diet. Therefore, smokers may need to take steps to soften this outer wall to allow nutrients and waste to pass back and forth. There are two very valuable nutrients that can help in this softening process, methylsulfonylmethane (commonly referred to as MSM) and essential fatty acids (omega-3 oils or fats). Both of these nutrients can be taken in supplement form and can help to soften the cell walls to allow for the intake and proper use of nutrients being sent to our cells. Nutrient entry and waste exit are also facilitated by the presence of certain minerals such as calcium and magnesium.

These minerals, calcium and magnesium, are just a few of the essential minerals that also determine whether our bodies are acidic or alkaline. Remember, an overly acidic body is caused by the consumption of too much saturated fat (red meat and dairy products), processed flour, processed sugar, and alcohol. The body becomes more alkaline, and thus more healthy, by eating less of these acidic foods and more vegetables and fruits. There are also excellent supplements that can help the body attain a proper acid alkaline balance, usually about 7.4 pH. One of these is Buffer pH™ from Vaxa International. Ordering guidelines are in the back of this book. (Test strips for measuring acid/alkaline levels can be purchased at any pharmacy.)

> The body becomes more alkaline, and thus, more healthy, by eating less of these acidic foods and more vegetables and fruits.

Conclusion

As you can see, the body is a complex set of systems and processes that must work together in an efficient and effective manner in order to achieve optimum health. For smokers, it may be easier to correct the faults in their digestive process than it is to quit their smoking habit. Selecting better food, chewing it properly, and taking a few supplements is not really that difficult, but it can have a tremendous impact on our health. Proper nutrient intake and digestion is the number one way for everyone to avoid illness and aging, but this is especially true for smokers who put their bodies at extra risk due to their habit. As the smoker's body becomes healthier, it is also very possible that the body's dependency on nicotine and other addictive chemicals will be lessened, thus giving the smoker an even better chance to kick his or her unfortunate addiction.

VII.   Nutritional Guidelines for Smokers

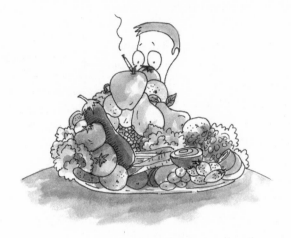

WE HAVE DISCUSSED THE MANY NEGATIVE ASPECTS of smoking from the 4,000 chemicals in each cigarette to all of the diseases that can be caused by smoking, such as heart disease and cancer. We have even touched on the various nutritional changes that can help smokers avoid these diseases by consuming more foods high in antioxidants such as fruits and vegetables. However, we have only scratched the surface in discussing the best foods for smokers to consume if they want to stimulate the body's natural cleansing process as well as ward off the diseases known to be caused by smoking.

Smoking has many dramatic impacts on the body, but eating the wrong foods can make these problems much worse. Therefore, we will start this discussion on nutrition with a list of foods that smokers should definitely avoid.

Foods to Avoid for Smokers
Junk Foods – This includes candy, potato chips, most fast food, and any food with a low nutrient value. These foods have empty calories, too much sugar, too much fat, and harmful chemicals that damage our cells much the same as nicotine and the other

chemicals in cigarettes do. Smokers don't need any extra cell-destroying products in their bodies.

Processed Foods – Foods that have been refined, as in the grinding of flour, or processed in some way, such as bleaching, are seriously devoid of nutrient value. The chemicals used in this processing, as well as the nutrients extracted, create foods that often do more harm than good in our bodies. They may taste good and provide some energy, but these are shallow benefits compared to the harm done as a result of the processing. Examples would be white bread, muffins, or pasta made from refined flour.

> The chemicals used in this processing, as well as the nutrients extracted, create foods that often do more harm than good in our bodies.

Saturated Fat – This is the bad fat found in most meat, dairy products, and other animal products or oils. This fat is the one that contributes to the build-up of plaque in our arteries and causes our cell walls to become hardened. Smokers can ill afford these additional health problems because they add to the negative influences of smoking. Tar and nicotine make our blood sticky and more vulnerable to plaque build-up as well as harming our cell walls.

Coffee and Tea – Reduce or eliminate most use of coffee or tea (except herbal teas) because caffeine is a stimulant in much the same way nicotine is a stimulant. Your nervous system does not need extra stimulation, which promotes the production of the negative hormone cortisol.

Alcohol – Some alcohol, such as a glass of red wine, has been shown to be helpful to smokers because of the antioxidants it contains, but hard liquor and beer should be avoided. Alcohol puts a strain on the liver, which is the body's primary cleansing organ. It does not need additional work or distractions as it attempts to cope with the toxins ingested by smoking.

Animal Protein – Animal protein is difficult to digest which slows down metabolism, is full of saturated fat, and, in some cases, contains chemicals and hormones. Processed meats (luncheon meat, bacon, smoked meat, and hot dogs) are the worst, but red meat, pork, and other meat from four-legged animals is usually filled with growth hormones, antibiotics, and other chemicals. These chemicals suppress your immune system and cause less efficient nutrient intake. Broiled fish is the best protein choice, especially wild salmon due to its high levels of omega-3 fats.

Peanuts – Any nut grown at or in the ground is subject to having a high level of fungus as well as high levels of fat. Examples would be peanuts and cashews. Choosing walnuts, almonds, Brazil nuts, and pecans is much wiser.

Soybean Products – Some scientists recommend the consumption of soybeans because they contain a very special form of nutrient called genisten, which has been shown to prevent cancer. However, there are other studies that indicate that soybeans contain certain enzyme inhibitors that can impede the nutrient uptake process. It might be wise to limit the intake of soybean products unless they are fermented.

Foods to Include for Smokers
The following foods have been shown to have the most beneficial impacts on the special health challenges facing smokers.

Cleansing Foods – Foods such as celery, watermelon, onions, garlic, and asparagus have proven cleansing properties, as do any foods with a high level of chlorophyll (i.e., dark green vegetables).

Antioxidant Foods – Most fruits and vegetables are good sources of antioxidants, but smokers should emphasize carrots, pumpkins, papaya, squash, yams, tomatoes, citrus fruit, spinach, and red and yellow peppers.

Anticancer Foods – Foods that are particularly helpful in preventing cancer include broccoli, brussels sprouts, cauliflower, cabbage, turnips, beets, alfalfa sprouts, apples, cherries, and grapes.

Hydrocarbon Destruction – Some foods are particularly good at neutralizing the hydrocarbons found in cigarette smoke; they include strawberries, grapes, and cherries, which contain high levels of ellagic acid, a phytochemical known to act against hydrocarbons.

Cell-Building Foods – To build healthy cells (RNA and DNA) the body needs foods such as milled cereal, wheat, oats, nuts, bran, red beans, eggs, lentils, and perhaps some lean organic chicken or turkey meat.

Water – The body needs clean water to help with cleansing and to avoid dehydration. Eight to ten glasses of spring or distilled water is desirable because tap water contains 500 different chemicals that are toxic to the body. Care should be taken to not overdo the consumption of distilled water since it can cause some leaching of calcium from the bones under certain conditions.

Calcium-rich Foods – Smoking inhibits the absorption of calcium by the body, which suggests the need to consume more foods with calcium to compensate for this loss. Milk is not the best source of calcium despite all of the ads about this purported benefit. Calcium can be obtained from broccoli, sardines, yogurt, and perhaps some quality dairy products such as goat's milk, goat's cheese, and organic skim milk. Pasteurized and homogenized cow's milk is not a very healthy product because it contains too many hormones and antibiotics. Some people are lactose intolerant, and homogenization pulverizes the fat molecules, allowing them to enter the bloodstream before proper digestion.

> Milk is not the best source of calcium despite all of the ads about this purported benefit.

This contributes to plaque build-up in the arteries.

Conclusion

This is just a small snapshot of the best foods for smokers, and there is, obviously, much more that could be presented on this topic. However, if smokers followed the guidelines offered in this chapter, as well as other parts of this book, they would realize 95% of the benefits they could obtain from eating better. The overall goal is to avoid foods with low nutrient value while consuming foods high in antioxidants and other nutrients needed by the body. For a more complete list see Appendix IV. The key is to maintain an alkaline body by eating a sufficient quantity of vegetables since they are the most alkaline foods available. Red meat, dairy products, sweets, and other fatty foods are acidic, and an acidic body is vulnerable to disease. It is not necessary to become obsessive about these eating guidelines, but most nutritionists agree consuming these healthy foods 80 or 90% of the time is highly recommended. The occasional sweet or other indulgence will likely not be harmful as long as a healthy diet is followed most of the time.

VIII.   The Importance of Supplementation

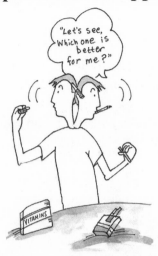

The Real Threat of Disease

MOST AMERICANS DO NOT THINK THEY ARE GOING to become ill
with a serious disease until the very day that it happens.
When the heart attack happens or the doctor utters those terrible
words "you've got cancer," the average person is very surprised
and thinks these things happen only to someone else. This is probably true of many smokers who should realize the potential danger
of their habit due to all of the publicity on this topic during the past
several years. The following facts fly directly in the face of this
prevailing public opinion.

- The Centers for Disease Control report that 50 years ago 10% of
  the population was chronically ill, and today that figure is over
  40%.
- One person dies each minute from cancer, and one in three
  Americans will die from some form of cancer.
- Heart disease causes one million deaths annually, and one in
  three men will develop some form of cardiovascular disease by
  the age of 60.
- Over half of women over 55 have some form of osteoporosis.

- More than 50 million Americans suffer from some form of arthritis.
- Diabetes affects more than 16 million people with several millions more having high blood sugar and being well on their way to diabetes. Diabetes is the leading cause of blindness, kidney disease, nerve disease, and amputations.
- About 43 million people suffer from high blood pressure.
- A new case of breast cancer is found every three minutes, and 75% of men over 60 will have a serious problem with their prostate.

These are very serious statistics that are reported on a regular basis, and yet a majority of people choose to ignore them and persist in the belief that it just won't happen to them. The patterns of poor health habits and behavior are firmly entrenched in our culture as can be seen by the following additional statistics.

- The percentage of overweight adults in the U.S. has reached an all time high of 63%, and 30% of children are overweight.
- Obesity cost our country over $60 billion last year in terms of the health consequences of being overweight (diabetes, heart disease, etc.).
- The Centers for Disease Control found in a recent survey that only 1% of Americans meet the minimum daily requirements for nutritional adequacy.
- Many people continue to use tobacco even though it has been clearly shown that smokers have a 70% greater overall mortality rate from disease than nonsmokers.
- Less than one in six Americans get even the minimum aerobic exercise necessary to keep their heart healthy.

When someone loses their good health their whole life changes for the worse. Disease is a serious distraction in our lives and drains us of time, money, energy, and the ability to perform many desirable activities. Over 50% of all personal bankruptcies are due, at least in part, to medically related expenses.

How do poor health and disease happen?

We don't start out each day trying to become less healthy, and yet many of the choices we make, or conditions we accept as normal, lead us in that very direction. Consider the following lifestyle and societal patterns.

- Stress continues to creep into our lives at work and at home.
- We eat on the run and get food where it is available.
- We eat too many fried foods and too many sweets.
- We give in to our addictions to caffeine in coffee and soft drinks.
- We skip meals when life just becomes too hectic.
- We eat foods that are grown in depleted soil.
- We eat foods that have been overtreated with pesticides.
- We eat foods that have been overcooked, processed, or microwaved.
- We eat too many carbohydrates (the simple processed variety).
- We don't take enough supplements to keep our bodies nourished.
- We don't drink enough water.
- Some of us drink too much alcohol.
- We don't pay attention to health patterns in our family (genes).
- We consume too many antibiotics, which deplete our immune system.
- We consume too many prescription drugs that aren't necessary.
- We don't exercise as much as we should.
- We don't practice relaxation and stress control every day.
- We allow harmful environmental conditions at work to persist.
- We often don't nurture our relationships as we should.
- We don't read enough about how to protect our health.

In other words, we go through life paying very little serious attention to the consequences of our unhealthy actions and then are shocked when we become ill. It would be more appropriate to be shocked if you did not become ill. There are some people

> "The key to longevity is to have a chronic disease and take good care of it."
>
> – Oliver Wendell Holmes, 1847

who even think that becoming ill early in life can actually be a blessing if it is not too serious and you take measures to correct it. In fact, this opinion has been known for many years. In 1847, Oliver Wendell Holmes was quoted as saying, *"The key to longevity is to have a chronic disease and take good care of it."*

This has certainly been true in my own case ever since I was diagnosed with a urinary tract problem over 25 years ago. By taking "good care of it," I have actually been able to become healthier with each passing year. Perhaps many smokers will seize this opportunity to become healthier and eventually become so healthy it will be easier for them to quit their own unfortunate habit.

My genes are good
I wish I had a dollar for every time I heard someone say, "I have good genes" and then that person became seriously ill within the next few years. If people read more about genes and disease, they would know that only 5% of cancers are passed on genetically and about 30% of all diseases can really be blamed on bad genes. That means that about 70% or more of our illnesses are due to things we do to ourselves, our so-called lifestyle choices.

In Jeffrey Bland's book *Genetic Nutritioneering*, even the apparent connection between our genes and the probability of becoming ill is questioned.

- People with defective genes can neutralize them to a significant degree by taking specific steps to overcome their inherited tendencies. Through diet, exercise, supplementation, meditation, and other natural health actions begun early in life, there is a very good chance that genetic health problems can be delayed or even totally avoided.
- Conversely, if you have wonderful genes, it is also possible for you to override them through a series of bad lifestyle choices. If you eat too many cholesterol-laden foods, don't exercise, and fill

your life with stress, you can have a heart attack even if none of your parents or grandparents had any type of heart disease. You are not immune from illness simply because your parents and grandparents lived to a ripe old age. Consider some of these changing conditions.

- Our parents had employment that was more stable and less stressful.
- Our forefathers were not subjected to the thousands of carcinogenic pollutants that we must contend with every day.
- Our parents' jobs required more physical labor. (This is a good thing.)
- Our parents and grandparents engaged in more physical recreational activities (no computers or television).
- Due to various scientific breakthroughs, like polio and smallpox vaccine, we are living longer than previous generations and are more susceptible to diseases related to old age such as Alzheimer's, Parkinson's, and some cancers.
- There was less junk food available to our parents and grandparents.

As an excuse for not paying more attention to our health, good genes is certainly not as acceptable as most people believe it is. However, it is only one of the many excuses put forward to avoid taking action to improve our health.

Everyone Will Die Sometime
This is another one of those casual comments people make in trying to dismiss the call for better diets, a cessation to smoking, or the elimination of some other bad habit that people don't want to give up. Consider the cases of a few people I have heard utter those words.

Case #1
T. F. is a friend of mine who lived the high life all through his twenties and thirties with plenty of parties, lots of alcohol, a few drugs,

a pretty bad diet, and no vitamins. He always said his father only made it to age 65 and that would be fine with him. In his late thirties, T. F. was informed he had Hepatitis C and cirrhosis of the liver. Now he must be on a special diet, take many drugs and vitamins, go to bed around 8 P.M. because he has no energy left, and live with constant pain and discomfort. He may live to age 65, but the last 25 years will not be what he was hoping for. He has humbly eaten the words he spoke as an impetuous young man.

Case #2

W. F. is also a friend of mine who would delight in teasing me about the many vitamins I was taking, the food I brought with me to replace the unhealthy fare he offered, my unwillingness to drink alcohol, and my insistence on exercising every day when, in his opinion, there were so many other more enjoyable things to do. When W. F. was about 40 he had his first bout of stomach ulcers, which he survived with the help of medication, and then thought he could just carry on as before. About five years later he had a more serious ulcer attack, which now included jaundice and a near death experience. I think this experience got his attention. Gradually, he has begun to change his diet, stop his consumption of alcohol, add vitamins and herbs to his daily routine, and read health journals about his multiple health problems. The quality of his life is a mere fraction of what it used to be as he must carefully watch everything he consumes, has much less energy than he used to, has lost much muscle mass, and has aged well beyond his actual years. Instead of teasing, now I get inquiries about how he can improve his condition and get back to good health.

There are so many similar stories of relatives who died at age 50 from cancer and young people in their twenties with Crohn's disease or fibromyalgia. There are even cases of parents asking what they can do about their teenager who has come down with Type II diabetes, which used to be a disease experienced mostly by people over 40. The sad part of these stories is that most of these health problems were totally avoidable.

How do supplements help?

Most of the health problems just discussed were due, in a large part, to the consumption of harmful foods and the insufficient intake of nutrients. It has also been clearly stated that eating healthy foods is the best way to get nutrients.

Supplements are not intended to replace the nutrients we get from our food, but rather add to or complement them. We still need to eat a healthy diet. For reasons previously stated, it is virtually impossible to get the vitamins, minerals, and enzymes we need from the foods that are available to us. And, the Recommended Daily Allowances (RDA) for vitamins and minerals are totally inadequate to meet the needs of the average person. They are the minimum requirements based on outdated research that has not been updated for political reasons. The explanation about the connection between the government's dietary and vitamin guidelines and the special interests of the medical establishment, the drug industry, and the food industry has already filled many books. The main point is that many progressive scientists and doctors have come to the conclusion that supplementation is very necessary and should be done at an optimal level as opposed to a minimal level. This is especially true for smokers who want to become healthier. Here is some of their reasoning.

> **Supplementation is very necessary and should be done at an optimal level as opposed to a minimal level.**

- Pollutants and other toxic substances invade our bodies every day, and we call these substances free radicals. If we don't get enough antioxidants (vitamins A, C, E, selenium, etc.), these free radicals will cause disease to occur.
- Our cells are replaced on a regular basis, some every few days (skin, stomach, etc.) or every few months (more dense body parts). If we do not eat right, and supplement, we will replace old cells with inferior new cells leading to premature aging and disease.
- Without the right nutrient levels, we reduce the body's ability to

produce various natural chemicals and hormones that perform vital functions like keeping our heart beating, allowing us to have sexual relations, or keeping our brain in good working order.

- Without the right enzymes, minerals, and vitamins, our food cannot be properly digested, which means nutrients cannot reach our cells or waste cannot be properly removed.

- Without a sufficient level of vitamins and minerals, our immune system becomes depressed, and we are unable to kill the various germs and bacteria that invade our bodies every day.

- Once we do succumb to some disease, it is possible for various supplements, including herbal remedies, to help us recover. (For example, milk thistle is an herb commonly used to support people with some form of liver disease.)

- As was previously stated, it is even possible to neutralize or overcome genetic tendencies for certain diseases with various supplements. The best example of this is heart disease.

A study by Pracon, Inc. of Reston, Virginia, indicated that if every American took 400 international units of vitamin E every day, health costs would be reduced by $8.7 billion per year. Most of the savings would be caused by a reduction of days spent in the hospital by more than 500,000 days per year. The equally amazing aspect of this example is that the benefits of vitamin E for the heart were identified over 50 years ago by Evan Shute, M.D. of London, Ontario. It has taken the medical community and the federal government over 50 years to admit to the benefits identified by Dr. Shute in his clinical research. How many lives have been lost, how many unnecessary drugs have been consumed, and how many unnecessary operations have been performed due to this stubborn resistance to the benefits of this one vitamin? How many billions of dollars have been wasted? A recent study suggested that vitamin E may cause health problems at high levels, but this flies in the face of hundreds of studies proving the benefits of vitamin E. And a closer examination of this study has revealed many flaws, which call into question the negative results from taking vitamin E.

Another tragic case of the medical community ignoring valuable scientific findings involved the work of Dr. Gilmore McCauley, who, 39 years ago, identified the importance of folic acid in the regulation of homocysteine metabolism. If doctors had listened to his research, over 1.5 million lives could likely have been saved instead of lost to diseases such as spina bifida, stroke, depression, Downs syndrome, colon cancer, and breast cancer. Aren't doctors supposed to prevent disease and do no harm?

What Are Vitamins?
Supplements are composed of vitamins, minerals, enzymes, and herbs, which "supplement" the foods we eat. The word vitamin comes from the Latin word vita, which means life. Vitamins were only discovered about one hundred years ago, although many scientists had suspected that there must be special substances that allowed the body to grow and protect itself from various germs and other toxins. The problems involved in getting enough vitamins from the food we eat has been discussed previously, but it is worth repeating that less than 1% of the population gets all of the vitamins, minerals, and enzymes they need for normal cell growth and pro-

> Of all recommendations in this book for improving the health of smokers, none is more important than taking supplements, other than quitting smoking.

tection. Smokers are particularly vulnerable to vitamin depletion because their habit either destroys vitamins in the body, such as vitamin C, or requires more of a particular vitamin due to the stress smoking places on the body. The lungs' need for vitamin A is an example of this increased vitamin requirement for smokers. Understanding how some of the key vitamins work in our body can help to encourage people, especially smokers, to take more vitamins as a way to protect their health. In fact, of all the recommendations in this book for improving the health of smokers, none is more important than taking supplements, other than quitting smoking.

Specific Supplements for Smokers

There are certain supplements that should be taken on a regular basis by practically everyone, because it is virtually impossible to get enough of certain nutrients from the food we eat. These supplements are listed in Appendix V and can serve as a general guideline for what supplements to take. However, among this list there are some supplements that are especially crucial for smokers because they help to offset or mitigate the negative impacts of smoking on the body's biochemistry. There are also some supplements that are not on this general list that should be added because of their special and proven ability to help smokers. Each of these smoker friendly supplements will be reviewed with some explanation about why they are so important for smokers.

Curcumin – This herb gets special consideration for smokers because it is recognized as one of the main reasons why Japanese men get cancer at a rate of one-half that of American men while smoking twice as much. It is consumed in the form of the spice known as turmeric, which is part of the ginger family. Curcumin has antioxidant properties that go well beyond the neutralizing of free radical toxins inhaled by smokers. Curcumin actually intercepts the pathways of cancer cells by also disrupting the attempts of any cancer cells to move from one part of the body to another. Curcumin is being studied by the National Institutes of Health for many other benefits including anti-atherosclerotic, anti-inflammatory, anti-viral, anti-fungal, and immune modulating effects (500-1,000 mg/day is recommended).

Vitamin C – Smokers destroy between 25 and 50 milligrams of vitamin C with every cigarette they smoke. This is not good because vitamin C is needed by the adrenal glands to synthesize hormones needed by the body for many reasons. Vitamin C is also a powerful antioxidant that scavenges free radicals that are plentiful in cigarette smoke (4,000 chemicals in each cigarette). The many and dramatic negative impacts of smoking on the body have been previously covered, and vitamin C can play a major role in preventing and minimizing this cellular damage (3,000-6,000 mg per day of vitamin C with bioflavonoids is recommended with dosages taken every four hours in order to keep enough vitamin C in your system at all times).

Pycnogenol – Pycnogenol is a powerful antioxidant found in foods such as grape seeds. This special nutrient helps boost the body's production of vitamin E and glutathione, which are strong scavengers of free radicals such as nitric oxide and hydroxyl radical. These free radicals are especially dangerous because they directly attack our DNA. There is another important benefit in pycnogenol's ability to control platelet aggregation, which is a major factor in the development of arterial plaque leading to strokes and/or heart disease. Pycnogenol is 500% better in this anti-platelet aggregation than aspirin, which is often touted as a leading "natural" blood-thinning agent. Unfortunately, aspirin can also cause bleeding ulcers and gastrointestinal distress, which pycnogenol does not. Pycnogenol also prevents the oxidation of LDL cholesterol, protects our artery lining, reduces inflammation, increases natural killer cell production, may prevent Alzheimer's disease, and protects our skin from ultraviolet radiation (50-100 mg/day is recommended).

Coenzyme Q10 – There are ongoing debates about whether Co Q10 is a vitamin or a ubiquinone (a word you may not have heard before). Ubiquinone is actually a new word that combines ubiquitous, meaning that Co Q10 is found in every cell in the body (all 60 trillion of them), and quinone, which is a biological chemical responsible for creating energy (which Co Q10 does in every cell). Co Q10 aids in the flow of oxygen to the brain, protects the heart tissue, and acts as an antioxidant to protect the cells of our lungs. Co Q10 should be taken with coenzyme A because they support each other (200-400 mg/day is recommended).

Vitamin E – This vitamin is one of the most important antioxidants because of its ability to protect the cells and organs that are damaged by cigarette smoke. Sometimes vitamins like vitamin E team up with selenium to detoxify certain metals in our bodies. Another toxin in tobacco smoke is nitrogen dioxide, which is converted into various carcinogens (cancer agents). Some studies have shown the ability of gamma tocopherol (a form of vitamin E) to neutralize nitrogen dioxide thus protecting smokers from lung cancer. Vitamin E also protects the heart and brain by reducing blood platelet aggregation, keeping arteries soft and flexible as well as destroying free radicals. It is highly advisable to consume a mixture of alpha, beta, delta, and gamma tocopherols rather than the cheaper formulation of vitamin E, which contains only alpha tocopherols. The benefit of the mixed blend is definitely worth the extra cost (400 iu/day is recommended).

Vitamin B Complex – The B vitamins are extremely important to the health of every person, especially smokers. The primary B vitamins include B1, B2, B3, B6, B12, biotin, folic acid, and pantothenic acid. The B vitamins are often associated with the maintenance of a healthy nervous system, because nerve cells require high doses of B vitamins in order to function properly. Smokers often use smoking to "control" their nerves or their "stress," but B vitamins can do a much better and safer job on this count. These vitamins also keep cellular enzyme levels high, which supports the growth of new cells. Smokers suffer from premature aging of internal and external cells, which can be minimized by taking regular doses of a wide range of B vitamins (100 mg/day of a B complex is recommended along with 1,000 mcg/day of Vitamin B12 and 400 mcg/day of folic acid).

Beta-carotene (Vitamin A) – There is some controversy over the desirability of smokers taking beta-carotene due to a Finnish study that showed an increased risk of cancer for smokers who took beta-carotene. However, examinations of this study have found numerous flaws, and there are many other studies over the past 20 years that show the clear benefits of beta-carotene and vitamin A in the prevention and treatment of lung cancer. Cells in the lungs need vitamin A to remain healthy, and beta-carotene is a precursor to vitamin A, which means it helps the body to produce as much as it needs. Vitamin A taken directly can be toxic in very large doses although that amount is extremely high (over 20,000 iu's). Many doctors recommend that their smoking patients take both vitamin A and beta-carotene because beta-carotene conversion occurs in the intestine and can be somewhat sluggish. Therefore, taking a preformed vitamin A may be more effective in the direct protection of the membranes in the lungs than beta-carotene, which has good general antioxidant capabilities (5,000-10,000 iu/day of vitamin A and 25,000-50,000 iu/day of beta-carotene is recommended).

Alpha Lipoic Acid – Alpha lipoic acid is not a vitamin because the body does produce a little on its own (vitamins are nutrients not produced by the body). However, as we age we produce less and less of this very important nutrient, and smoking increases our need for it due to the oxidative stress that occurs with smoking. Smoking also disrupts the production and transportation of glutathione in the body that can be the beginning of diseases such as diabetes, stroke, heart disease, cataracts, and cancer. Alpha lipoic acid has been proven effective in the prevention and treatment of each of these diseases and has the unique ability to balance deficiencies of vitamins E and C in the body. Smokers are vulnerable to all of these diseases at a much higher rate than the general population and therefore should use alpha lipoic acid as one of the ways to minimize the likelihood of these diseases beginning (100-200 mg/day is recommended).

Zinc – Zinc is a mineral with very strong antioxidant capabilities. It is especially helpful to smokers because of its ability to prevent cadmium levels from increasing in the body. Cadmium is one of the more dangerous toxins in cigarette smoke, which depletes and replaces the body's reserve of zinc in the liver and kidneys. This has a dramatically negative impact on our immune system, and supplementing with zinc can reduce this negative influence (30-40 mg/day is recommended).

Inositol – This vitamin helps prevent hardening of the arteries which is a specific condition encouraged by smoking. It also is important in the formation of lecithin and the metabolism of fat and cholesterol, which is impeded by smoking. A deficiency of inositol can lead to irritability and mood swings, which also occur as smokers go through withdrawal on their way to cessation. Inositol also combines with vitamin B in the body to provide a source of energy (100 mg/day).

Glutamine – This amino acid is very important because it can easily pass the blood-brain barrier where it is converted to glutamic acid, which is essential for cerebral function. It helps maintain a proper acid/alkaline balance in the body as well as being a building block for the synthesis of RNA and DNA. Glutamine helps clear ammonia from brain tissue and muscles, which can lower the impact of stress on the body as well as decrease craving for things like sugar, alcohol, and nicotine (900-1000 mg/day).

GABA – Gamma-aminobutyric acid is an amino acid that is formed from glutamic acid and, along with inositol and niacin-amide, helps to prevent stress-related messages from reaching the motor centers of the brain. This is crucial for smokers who are trying to replace cigarettes as a means of calming their nerves and managing stress (1,000 mg/day).

Other Helpful Supplements for Smokers
There are some other supplements beyond those on the above list that should be seriously considered by smokers due to their proven ability to help reduce the negative consequences of smoking.

Quercitin – This bioflavonoid mediates allergic and inflammatory responses in the body and reduces the damage induced by tobacco on membranes in the air passageways (1,200 mg/day).

Glutathione – Stimulates the production of interleukin 1 (especially in older people, above 50), which reduces inflammation and fights infection. Also, it promotes lymphocyte proliferation helping immune cell production (50-100 mg/day).

Maitake mushroom extract – Inhibits carcinogens in the body and protects against the spread of cancer through the lungs (1,000-1,500 mg/day).

Selenium – Helps protect cells from oxidative cell damage. Often taken with vitamin E (200 mcg/day).

Lycopene – Proven most effective in the treatment of prostate, lung, and stomach cancers as well as some evidence in the prevention of heart disease. This is the nutrient in tomatoes that is part of the carotenoid family (15-20 mg/day).

Omega-3 fatty acids – This essential fatty acid is found in certain fish (salmon) and flax seeds. It helps cells to stay soft and flexible thus allowing nutrients in and waste out. Omega-3 oils also protect brain cells, our heart, and our joints as well as preventing blood clotting (1,000-5,000 mg/day).

MSM – (methylsulfonylmethane) – MSM is found in fruits, vegetables, red meat and grains and has been shown to protect cell membranes in order to encourage proper cellular formation. May help prevent cancer (500 mg/day).

Garlic – Garlic is a very powerful anti-viral, anti-bacterial, anti-fungal plant (herb), which does everything from lowering blood pressure and cholesterol to reducing blood sugar and preventing cancer (600 mg/day – ensure allicin yield of at least 4,000 mcg).

Astragalus – This powerful herb is one of the most effective herbal medicines used in China for over 2,000 years. It is being studied by the National Cancer Institute for the prevention and treatment of breast and lung cancer (500 mg/day).

When To Take Supplements

Taking supplements is not as easy as just putting them in a container and taking them all at once in the morning to get it out of the way. Supplements are nutrients with specific properties that should be taken at certain times and in certain sequences. If you are going to spend the money to improve your health with supplements, *please take the time to do it right*. Here are some easy-to-follow guidelines. Once you get used to a routine, it will become second nature to you like brushing your teeth or combing your hair.

1. Generally it is advisable to take supplements with meals and to spread them out over the day. For example, when you take vitamin C, take 500-1,000 mg at a time about every four hours. Vitamin C only stays active for about that long, and your body can only use about 500 mg at a time. Your body can handle much larger doses if you are sick, or have high levels of free radicals.

2. Take fat-soluble vitamins (A, E, and K) with fatty foods such as salmon, almond butter, or some other healthy fat. This will greatly assist assimilation.

3. To assist in overall supplement assimilation, it may be advisable to take a probiotic (acidophilus) in the morning about 20 minutes before breakfast to ensure there is enough friendly bacteria in your intestines. A digestive enzyme prior to each meal or some raw vegetable will also aid digestion, especially as you get older (i.e., over age 50).

4. Vitamin B supplements should be taken at the same time, if possible, because they seem to work better when they are all present in the body.

5. Calcium, magnesium, and potassium should be taken during the day but at least one dose should be taken at bedtime because that is when the body balances its pH (acid/alkaline balance). If these minerals are in your bloodstream while you sleep, the body is less likely to steal calcium from your bones or magnesium from your muscles in order to help your body to become less acidic and more alkaline.

6. When eating foods with cholesterol (eggs, lobster, meat, etc.), it is advisable to take a lecithin capsule (1,000 mg); this will help to neutralize the bad cholesterol.

7. You should double your antioxidant intake (vitamin C, vitamin E, selenium, beta-carotene, alpha lipoic acid, etc.) or increase other supplements under these circumstances:

• More antioxidants when exercising strenuously. This releases free radicals from your lymph nodes and creates more free radicals in your cells.
• More antioxidants when receiving x-rays or radiation. This produces more free radicals.
• More antioxidants when taking antibiotics. This weakens your immune system and kills friendly bacteria.
• More antioxidants when receiving chemotherapy. This dramatically weakens your immune system.
• More antioxidants when in a polluted environment. This increases exposure to free radicals.
• More antioxidants when you are on heart medicine. Especially take more Co Q10 which is depleted by many heart medicines (statins).
• More antioxidants when you are under stress because more free radicals are produced. Take extra B vitamins.
• More antioxidants when you are exposed to colds or flu viruses. Your immune system needs a boost. Take extra garlic, echinacea, zinc, and astragalus as well.
• More antioxidants when you eat a lot of sweets (which you

shouldn't). This lowers your immune system and feeds germs.

- At least one day a week give yourself a rest from most supplements so your body does not become too dependent on them and excess amounts can be flushed from the body or used up.

Supplement Cautions
As a general rule the supplements covered in this book are safe for consumption by a vast majority of the population. There are some common guidelines that can help to ensure the continued safe use of these valuable nutritional supplements.

1. Pregnant women should always consult with a qualified holistic medical doctor before using any supplements because of their sensitive condition.

2. People who are on any kind of medication, including chemotherapy, should check with a holistic medical doctor. Some doctors still recommend against taking antioxidants during chemotherapy, but this has been proven not to be good advice. Find a doctor who is in touch with the latest research because the risks are too great not to get it right.

3. Vitamin A – More than 20,000 iu's per day can eventually lead to liver damage, hair loss, blurred vision and headaches.

4. Vitamin B6 – More than 400 mg per day can eventually affect nerves creating numbness in the mouth, hands, or legs.

5. Vitamin C – More than 10,000 mg per day can cause diarrhea. Take only bonded C (Ester C). (Diarrhea could be caused by a lesser amount in some people.)

6. Vitamin D – More than 1,000 iu's per day can cause calcium deposits that can interfere with muscle function, including the heart muscle.

7. Niacin – More than 2,000 mg per day can create liver problems, including jaundice. A flushed feeling, which is okay, can occur even with small doses.

8. Iron – More than 100 mg per day can interfere with the absorption of zinc leading to delays in healing, negative impacts on the immune system, or an increased risk of heart disease.

9. Beta-carotene – Synthetic forms can have a risk for smokers by actually increasing their risk of lung cancer according to one study. Use lower doses, under 50,000 iu's daily, and natural forms.

10. Calcium – Limit intake to less than 300 mg per day if you have kidney problems or hyperthyroidism.

11. Vitamin E – Avoid taking vitamin E if you are taking blood-thinning medication or taking aspirin on a daily basis.

12. Selenium – Don't exceed 1,000 mcg daily as some people have experienced loss of hair, teeth, or nails as well as dermatitis, upset stomach, and even paralysis.

All supplements should be taken under the watchful eye of a qualified health practitioner. However, everyone has the responsibility to also protect themselves by researching the potential negative impacts of any product. To check for possible reactions or contraindications you can go on the internet to www.alternative-dr.com and look up any supplement or prescription drug. This will provide a good backup for opinions received from health care providers if there is any inconsistency.

All Supplements Are Not Equal
Please do not make the mistake of thinking that all supplements are the same, even if a misinformed medical doctor tells you this.

Remember when they told you that taking vitamins was just creating expensive urine? They were wrong then, and they are wrong on this count also. There is a definite difference between the quality of products produced by various companies. In a new publication entitled *Comparative Guide to Nutritional Supplements*, over 500 supplements were compared for bio-availability and a number of other quality criteria. The companies that scored the highest were the ones following the same kind of quality standards required by the FDA of drug companies. Vaxa International exceeds these quality standards.

It is false economics, and bad for your health, to pick a cheaper or more heavily advertised brand, because you may be throwing your money away and not helping your health very much. As a general rule, the cheaper brands are less effective because these companies are not involved in basic research or using a very rigorous quality control process. You may pay more for quality products but actually get much more value for your money. Some cheaper products only assimilate at a level of 10-20%, while the more expensive ones may assimilate at 80% or higher. Spending even two or three times as much in these cases is definitely worth it. It's your health we are talking about. How much is it worth?

> **You may pay more for quality products but actually get much more value for your money.**

Are Your Vitamin Deficiencies Showing?

If we are not getting the vitamins we need, our bodies do not function as well as they otherwise should. Long before any disease presents itself, there are subtle warning signs to let us know that our intake of certain nutrients may not be adequate. These may be minor aches, discomforts, or inconveniences (sometimes called "subclinical" conditions) that do not show up on laboratory tests. By studying such symptoms in detail, we can usually get a very good picture of which vitamins may be lacking. A list of common vitamin deficiencies are shown in Appendix VI.

Summary

Keeping track of the desirable supplements and taking them on a consistent basis can be a real challenge even for the very motivated smoker. To make this important responsibility easier a new product has been developed that includes all of the primary nutrients needed by smokers who are trying to become healthier so they can eventually stop smoking. This new formulation has been developed by Vaxa International with the assistance of qualified biochemists and incorporates all of the key supplements recommended in this book. The list of ingredients can be seen in Appendix VII, and this product can be ordered using the guidelines in the back of this book (Appendix I).

> Long before any disease presents itself, there are subtle warning signs to let us know that our intake of certain nutrients may not be adequate.

IX. The Importance of Exercise

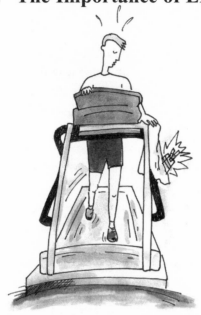

EXERCISE IS CRITICAL TO EVERYONE'S HEALTH but even more so for smokers. Lungs are the focal point of most health issues for smokers because this is where the smoke and its chemical cocktail are consumed for redistribution throughout the body. Lung cancer and other lung-related diseases are the most frequent health problems experienced by smokers. Keeping the lungs in the best possible working condition is one of the most important considerations for people who want to become healthier so they can eventually quit smoking.

There may be a misperception among many smokers that smoking is a serious limitation to being physically active, and while that can be true, it is not always the case. Several years ago I was involved with a ballet group and was shocked to learn that a majority of the ballerinas were heavy smokers. After discussing this situation with several of the dancers, I learned that the smoking served two main purposes, at least in their minds. The first involved their need to stay slim and their belief that smoking suppressed their appetite. The second had to do with stress management, since learning new dance routines every week was stressful and the artistic director had a harsh and autocratic style. Smoking, in their opinion, allowed them to stay calm and stay slim. What was truly amazing was the ability of these dancers to perform very strenuous dance routines for hours at a time without any apparent negative impact due to smoking. How were they able to smoke and still perform at the level of a world-class athlete? This shouldn't be possible according to all of the so-called experts on athletic performance.

The key to this high level of physical performance for these smoking dancers was the eight-hour exercise program they participated in six days per week. The lungs didn't really have much of a chance to become clogged or damaged because they were constantly working and expelling most of the harmful chemicals. There was also an excretion of toxins through the continuous sweating that the dancers were doing. Add to this the high protein and vegetable diets some of them were on and you can see how they were able to stay so healthy in spite of their bad habit.

Of course, the average person could never expect to devote eight hours a day to exercising, but that doesn't mean that a smoker can't get considerable benefit from a regular exercise program. Recently a friend who smokes started walking just 30 minutes every day and noticed a big change in her energy levels in less than two weeks. She was a very heavy smoker at the time, one and a half packs per day, and was able to cut back to 10 cigarettes a day using a combination of walking, better diet, and some supplements. Whereas she used to get very tired walking less than 100 feet, now she was able to go for walks on shopping trips for long distances without needing to rest. As her health continues to improve, she should continue to reap many other health benefits. She is already experiencing fewer headaches and afternoon energy crashes as a result of the few changes mentioned above.

Find an Exercise You Like
Everyone realizes the importance of exercise and yet many people are unable to sustain a regular exercise program. There are many factors that contribute to this difficulty in sustaining an exercise program, including time pressures, the expense involved, lack of energy, and lack of desire, just to mention a few of the most common reasons given by smokers. All of these basic exercise barriers can be overcome if you can find an exercise you really like.

In one case, a smoker had enjoyed dancing earlier in his life so he decided to join an adult dance class. The classes not only took his mind off his desire to smoke, they actually helped to reduce that desire for several hours after the lesson was over. In this case, exercise served many valuable purposes for this lucky smoker. First, it interrupted his normal pattern of smoking, which psychologists say is one of the keys to stopping a habit like smoking. Second, it provided the necessary exercise to clean out his lungs as well as expand his arteries, which reduces the build-up of plaque. Finally, it reduced his overall desire to smoke for several hours. This same group of benefits can be gained by almost any type of light aerobic exercise such as biking, swimming, walking, volleyball, or rebounding on a mini-trampoline.

Take it Easy to Start
It is advisable to start any exercise program slowly, especially if you have been inactive for any length of time. A visit to the doctor wouldn't hurt so you can get clearance to begin your program without the worry of complications. Starting slow and building your program gradually is important, especially because your mind may still think you are a young and athletic person. Many weekend athletes come home with injuries because they forgot, or didn't realize, what kind of condition they were in. Smoking actually destroys vitamin C, which is responsible for building connective tissue in our bodies (collagen). That means smokers are even more vulnerable to injuries than the nonsmoking weekend

athlete. That is precisely why I recommend that smokers consume extra amounts of vitamin C, both in the foods they eat and in supplements. Remember to stretch before and after exercising because your muscles need that limbering up in order to perform better and without injury.

Replace Some Other Activity
Many smokers have found it helpful to replace a typical smoking time with some type of exercise. At coffee breaks, or just after eating, try to go for a walk (without your cigarettes), and you may find there are many benefits to be realized. As in the earlier dancer's story, such pattern-breaking changes can help reduce the number of cigarettes smoked, provide some aerobic benefit, and reduce the desire to smoke. It should also be mentioned that studies have shown the addictive urge to smoke lasts from three to five minutes for most people. Getting past that short craving period can be helped by the diversion of exercise.

> Many smokers have found it helpful to replace a typical smoking time with some type of exercise.

Watching television may be a relaxing experience, but many people are relaxing a little too much. Resolve to give up 30 or 60 minutes of television in the evening to play softball with your kids or go for a bike ride around the neighborhood. Those are enjoyable experiences but can only take the place of smoking or sedentary activities if you resolve to make that change. Holding yourself accountable is an important part of following through on your exercise program.

Some Beginning Ideas
Doing an exercise or activity you already know and like is certainly an advantage, but some people may find that starting something completely new is the best approach for them. Some suggestions might include:

Yoga – This will not only stretch underutilized muscles, it will also help you to learn some valuable breathing and stress reduction techniques. Yoga can be an excellent beginning activity for the smoker who has not been very active for several years. In addition to the above-mentioned benefits, yoga can teach you about "mind control" and the ability to visualize desirable changes in your life. This is especially true when yoga is combined with meditation, which is often the case. Make certain that you search for the right yoga class for you by speaking with the instructors, as well as some of the existing participants.

Tai Chi – This is another excellent beginning activity for people wanting to start an exercise program because, like yoga, it can be as easy or as strenuous as you want it to be. Some poses are very gentle and stress balancing and centering, while others work certain muscle groups and encourage special breathing techniques. As with yoga, it is important to find the tai chi class that suits your needs in terms of timing, location, instructor, and participants. Who knows, after you have mastered many of the tai chi elements, you may want to move on to some of the more physical martial arts such as karate or tai kwon do.

Weight Lifting – Weight lifting, or any resistance training, has the advantage of potentially increasing fitness in terms of strength as well as aerobic fitness. There is also the advantage of being able to start very slowly and build your exercise program gradually as your body and conditioning permits. The aerobic part of resistance can be achieved by increasing the number of repetitions and decreasing the resting time between exercises. Increased resistance can be achieved by decreasing the number of repetitions and increasing the amount of weight used. Resistance training programs "do not" always need to happen at a fitness center, although some people seem unable to motivate themselves to work out at home and need the encouragement of others being around them. Having a good trainer to help design your program is very important, and some people, who can afford it, may wish to work with a trainer on a regular basis. One of the keys to the success of resistance training, or any exercise program, is consistency. This is often difficult because of the time commitment and the potential for exercising to become boring. That is why it is strongly advised that you vary your program every week or two at a minimum. The importance of using a good trainer at the beginning cannot be stressed strongly enough. One of the main reasons people are not able to sustain their exercise program is their lack of ability to get results. This is usually because they are doing the wrong exercises in the wrong sequence or they're using poor technique. Another reason is a poor diet. Without proper nutrition exercise programs are not only a waste of time, they may actually do more harm than good.

The Value of Exercising

A scientist once said that exercise is ten times more powerful, in terms of its health benefits, than the strongest vitamin or mineral supplement known to mankind. If someone could bottle exercise, they could become a very rich person. The benefits of exercise to anyone, including smokers, are many.

Detoxification – One of the biggest benefits of exercise for smokers is the improved ability to rid the body of toxins. Each cigarette has over 4,000 chemicals in it, and these toxins build up in the lungs, the heart, in other organs, and in fat cells. This is one of the leading causes of the heart disease, cancers, and other diseases experienced by smokers. Exercise helps to rid the body of these toxins through sweat as well as the motion of the lymphatic system, which is the storage place for most toxins before they are sent to the liver for processing. This stimulated release of toxins from lymph glands

> A scientist once said that exercise is ten times more powerful, in terms of health benefits, than the strongest vitamin or mineral supplement known to mankind.

can actually overload the liver with excessive toxins and should be carefully monitored. Many doctors recommend that athletes use liver supportive supplements such as milk thistle or DMG in order to help the liver cope with these excess toxins. Smokers would be wise to add these supplements to their program in order to help their liver process the toxins released by exercising.

Earlier in this book a comprehensive detoxification product from Vaxa International was strongly recommended. Since our program encourages detoxification of the entire body, it is advisable to use a liver support supplement to help the liver cope with increased levels of toxins. Vaxa International has a complementary product designed specifically to work in cooperation with their detoxification product. This product is a scientifically designed liver cleansing and support product that should be used with this detoxification program. Guidelines for ordering this product appear in the back of this book (Appendix I).

Hormone Balance – Smokers often have too much cortisol in their systems, because this often harmful hormone is stimulated by smoking and released by messages from the brain to the adrenal gland. Exercising helps to produce positive hormones that can counter negative hormones in much the same way that yoga, tai chi, and meditation produce such positive hormones. There are thousands of hormones produced by our bodies to help with various functions such as our sexual activities, our immune system, and every other system. Exercise helps to keep these hormones in balance, which is crucial for smokers who seem to suffer from swings in their hormone levels due to the stimulation of nicotine and the other strong chemicals in tobacco.

Oxygen Distribution – Every cell needs oxygen to reproduce, produce energy, get rid of waste, and perform its intended functions. People who don't exercise are deficient in their oxygen levels and thus suffer from premature aging and cell deterioration. Smokers are even more oxygen deprived because tar and nicotine take the place of oxygen in blood cells that travel throughout the body to deliver nutrients and oxygen as well as remove wastes. By exercising, smokers are forcing more oxygen into this equation, forcing out tar and nicotine, and greatly increasing the opportunity for cells to get the oxygen they so desperately need.

> By exercising, smokers are forcing more oxygen into this equation, forcing out tar and nicotine, and greatly increasing the opportunity for cells to get the oxygen they so desperately need.

Metabolism Improved – Exercise increases our body's metabolism, which means fat is burned for energy, muscle is formed which is more efficient at burning calories, and our digestive system moves a little quicker. Exercise increases the production and efficiency of insulin receptors on our cells. This improves the burning of glucose and insulin at the cellular level thus helping to avoid weight gain and stress on our pancreas. The cell replacement and repair process is expedited when our metabolism is working efficiently. Exercise increases our body temperature, which also causes many germs and bacteria to die because they don't like increased body temperature. Increased metabolism helps to keep our weight under control, which is often a complaint of smokers who are cutting back on their smoking or quitting.

Feel Good Stimulators – Some of those positive hormones previously mentioned are endorphins that are the feel good hormones that improve our moods and energy levels. Other good hormones include serotonin and melatonin, which are also stimulated with exercise and can help encourage better sleep patterns, fewer headaches, and a host of other mind-body benefits.

Disease Avoidance – Perhaps the most significant benefit of exercise for smokers is all of the nasty diseases they will be able to potentially avoid including heart disease, cancer, diabetes, osteoporosis, and more. There is no guarantee that these diseases will not occur just with the addition of exercise, but certainly the probability will be greatly reduced. Other factors must always be considered, including genetics, nutrition, and other lifestyle factors. Many scientific studies have proven that even light exercise can greatly reduce the risk of many diseases for the general public as well as for smokers.

It Doesn't Take Much

In a study by Dr. Steven Blair, published in the *Journal of the American Medical Association,* it was confirmed that a little exercise goes a long way. Tests were conducted on 10,224 men and 3,120 women over an eight-year period. In terms of death rates per 10,000 people, the sedentary, or virtually no exercise, group had the highest death rate at 64/10,000, while the group that walked 30 minutes every day had a death rate of only 25.5/10,000 or less than half the death rate of the sedentary group. The amazing outcome of this study revealed that men who ran 30-40 miles per week didn't fare much better. Other studies have produced similar results, which is why the 30-minute walk is now considered an acceptable minimum standard for an exercise program. (A brisk walk is best.)

Some Exercise Cautions

There are cautions that should be understood for anyone starting an exercise program.

- **After Eating** – Blood is needed in your stomach for at least an hour after eating. Then light exercise is fine. Strenuous exercise should probably be avoided for two hours after eating.
- **After Smoking** – Try to exercise well after smoking (30 minutes or more) because smoking constricts your arteries and limits oxygen flow to your muscles. In fact, try to replace your normal smoking times with exercise in order to break the smoking pattern.
- **Hot or Cold Weather** – In both cases your cardiovascular system is under additional stress. In hot weather avoid dehydration and overexercising. In cold weather be certain to stretch in the warm-up and the cool-down periods to avoid cramping.
- **After Drinking Alcohol** – Exercising within a few hours of consuming alcohol can encourage irregular heartbeat due to the heart stimulating effect of alcohol and exercise. Drinking after exercise is less of a problem, but be certain your heart has returned to its normal level before consuming alcohol.
- **Altitude** – Higher altitude causes less oxygen to be available for your lungs. Decreasing the intensity and duration of exercise is probably advisable when exercising at high altitudes.
- **Illness or Injury** – Exercising when ill or injured is not usually advisable, even for trained athletes. Illness lowers your immune function and exercising can make your illness worse. The same is true of an injury because your body needs all of the available energy for the healing process.
- **Medications** – Many medications can create problems for those who exercise. Check with your physician before starting an exercise program if you are on any type of medication.

The following chart contains some of the most commonly used medications, as well as the exercise precautions that should be followed.

Conditions	Medications	Workout Warnings	RX for Exercise
Allergies, sinusitis	Diphenhydramine (Benadryl) or other antihistamines	May cause drowsiness or dizziness, impair coordination, or slow reaction time.	Avoid movements and equipment that will throw you off balance. Try seated cardio activities like indoor cycling and rowing, or equipment with handrails, like stairsteppers and elliptical trainers.
Depression	Sertraline (Zoloft), fluoxetine (Prozac, Sarafem)	May cause drowsiness, nausea, or stomach upset that usually resolves in a few weeks.	Avoid working out until your stomach settles. If the drowsiness continues, stick to seated cardio equipment such as indoor cycles and rowing machines.
Anxiety	Alprazolam (Xanax)	May make you you drowsy and affect your coordination. Side effects generally taper off in a few weeks.	Take a pass on complicated moves like highly choreographed dance and aerobics routines. Try seated cardio equipment until you've adjusted.

Conditions	Medications	Workout Warnings	RX for Exercise
Asthma	Theophyline (Uniphy)	May cause dangerous heart rate increases if you have high blood pressure or heart disease. Good choices for active people are albuterol (Proventil) and montelukast (Singulair).	Ask your doctor if an alternative would be appropriate. If necessary have her/him approve your workout and adjust your drug dosage. Avoid extreme heat and cold. Warm up for at least 10 minutes, then cool down gradually. Always keep your bronchodilator on hand.
Colds	Pseudoephedrine (Sudafed, Triaminic)	May raise your temperature and heart rate to risky levels if you work out in extreme heat, or have high blood pressure or heart disease.	Don't work out if you have an elevated temperature, severe congestion, or serious chronic health problems. Otherwise, drink water before, during, and after exercising. Scale back on workout length and intensity.

Conditions	Medications	Workout Warnings	RX for Exercise
Diabetes	Glyburide (Micronase), repaglinide (Prandin), insulin, and other medications that lower blood sugar.	Intense activity may cause fainting or dizziness. If you are insulin-dependent, ask your doctor about adjusting your dosage.	Never work out on an empty stomach; eat a high-carbohydrate, high-fiber snack, such as half an almond butter sandwich on multigrain bread, 30 to 60 minutes beforehand.

X. Natural Therapies for Smokers

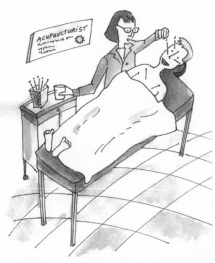

FOLLOWING THE THEORY THAT ANY SMOKER CAN become healthier without actually stopping their smoking, it is worthwhile to consider the many complementary or alternative therapies available to assist in this process. Most smoking cessation programs use some alternative or substitute for nicotine to help the body's physiological needs or various psychological techniques to overcome the habitual nature of smoking. Rarely do any of these programs attempt to make the body stronger or healthier as a way to help a person reduce his or her cravings. There are many therapies that can support not only the lungs, but also the many other parts of the body that can be negatively impacted by smoking. By counteracting the negative impacts of smoking with one or more of these therapies, a smoker can become healthier and thus avoid or at least minimize the short- and long-term consequences of smoking.

Breathing Techniques

For smokers it is obvious that the most compromised bodily function is usually breathing. The lungs become clogged with tar, nicotine, and other tobacco residue, which gradually reduces their ability to exchange carbon dioxide for oxygen. Blood is less able to deliver oxygen and nutrients to our cells or remove the waste products produced by our cells. Smokers tend to not exercise as much as they should because they have difficulty breathing, which allows the lungs to become even more clogged. If smokers can find a way to improve their breathing through proven breathing techniques, then more exercise would be feasible and the lungs could retain more of their important functions.

Most people, whether smokers or not, retain about 25% of the stale air in their lungs every time they exhale. This means that the lungs are only operating at 75% of their capacity and are unable to process the oxygen necessary for the body to function properly. This happens because most people only utilize one of the two possible methods of breathing. We can use either our chest only, our upper lung, or our entire diaphragm, which engages all of our lungs. The shallow breathing that uses only our chest muscles not only leaves stale air in the lungs, it can promote stress that can lead to anxiety, headaches, tiredness, heart disease, and even irritable bowel syndrome. For smokers these problems are exaggerated because they are also challenged by the pollutants added to this breathing equation.

Everyone, but especially smokers, should learn the techniques of deep breathing by practicing the following breathing exercises.

1. Sit in a comfortable and upright position while staying relaxed. Relaxation is one of the keys to diaphragm-based deep breathing.

2. Place one hand just under your rib cage and the other at the top of your chest. In deep breathing your lower hand will move in and out while your upper hand will not.

3. Once you have mastered the deep breathing technique, you should sit quietly and inhale slowly until you feel that your lungs are full and exhale just as slowly while maintaining very relaxed

and calming thoughts. Exhale completely so that the lungs are empty and then repeat this process several times. You may even want to close your eyes and picture some calming place or situation to help with your relaxation.

Dr. Andrew Weil promotes a similar technique that recommends four successive deep breaths until the lungs are full then holding your breath for the count of seven and then letting the air out in eight short bursts. The breathing in and out is done through the mouth.

There are also desirable techniques for breathing when you are walking or involved in other activities. When walking try to take two breaths in and as many as five breaths out. At first you may only be able to do two in and two out, but as your lung capacity improves, you should be able to increase the out breaths to three then four and finally five. This will allow you to replace your stale air on a regular basis and keep a good flow of oxygen and carbon dioxide to your cells. (Your body needs some carbon dioxide for certain functions such as digestion, circulation, and immune function.)

When the brain gets sufficient oxygen, it is encouraged to produce anti-stress hormones that counteract the stress hormones such as cortisol. This will be a very positive side benefit of the deep breathing exercises just explained.

Yoga
Some forms of yoga have been around for over 5,000 years and were originally developed as a way to improve a person's spiritual awareness. In North America, yoga is now practiced more for its physical benefits than its spiritual ones. Most forms of yoga incorporate gentle exercises and postures as well as breathing, meditation, relaxation, and diet. The general benefits include the toning of muscles, the strengthening of the spine, and improved suppleness or flexibility. For smokers there are definite benefits for practicing

yoga in terms of strengthening the respiratory muscles and toning of the lung tissues. Learning breath control can also help make the lungs less sensitive to allergens, which is a serious problem for many smokers. And finally, it should be understood that keeping the spine flexible and exercised allows the nerves coming out of the spinal column to keep the body's muscles and organs functioning properly. This combination of good nerves and muscles also contributes to the delivery of a good blood supply that ensures the delivery of oxygen and nutrients as well as the removal of wastes. Yoga can be a vitally important tool for smokers who want to become healthier even before they may be able to quit their smoking habit.

> If yoga can take the place of smoking in the control of stress, this may improve the smoker's ability to reduce or even quit his or her smoking habit.

Another benefit of practicing yoga is the improved ability to relieve and control stress and tension. This is especially valuable for smokers who often depend on smoking to help in the relief of stress or tension. If yoga can take the place of smoking in the control of stress, this may improve the smoker's ability to reduce or even quit his or her smoking habit.

There are many ways to learn the various yoga positions of which there are hundreds. Most people only practice the 20 positions that are the least difficult to perform. Joining a yoga class is the favorite method of learning for most people, but some people have purchased a book or video and even used television classes as a way to practice yoga. It is important to follow some basic guidelines because it is possible to do some positions the wrong way, which could pull or strain certain muscles. Some basic guidelines are as follows.

1. Start by wearing loose clothes and no shoes.
2. Using a mat of some kind on the floor is advisable.

3. Yoga should be practiced on an empty stomach.
4. Start by doing some basic stretches and deep breathing while lying on your back.
5. Never hurry or strain to achieve any position.
6. Keep your movements slow and graceful.
7. Most postures should be done in combination to stretch a muscle group in one direction and then in the opposite direction.
8. Remember that controlled deep breathing is an important part of any yoga position.

Yoga, like any exercise or lifestyle change, will only be beneficial if it is done properly and regularly. Having a regular routine is very helpful because it ensures consistency and gets the body used to certain rhythms in your life.

Meditation

Meditation is another technique for developing better breathing mechanics and capacity. It is based on thousands of years of experience believed to have started with an early Eastern religion such as Buddhism. When practiced effectively, meditation enables a person's mind to take complete control of many bodily functions such as breathing, heart rate, blood pressure, temperature, and even tolerance for pain. Some other beneficial physical changes, which are not as immediately noticeable as the above listed ones, include relaxed muscles, the alteration of brain waves, and the production of stress-reducing hormones.

For smokers, meditation can produce some very important health enhancements worthy of consideration. Muscles become relaxed around the air passages, which aids in the intake of oxygen and the expelling of carbon dioxide. This can lead to improved lung function and partial mitigation of the negative effects of smoking. Smoking tends to increase heart rate and blood pressure as well as stimulate the release of stress related hormones, and meditation can help to reduce some of these problems.

Meditation seems to be more popular with women than men because it is perceived as an unmanly or non-macho thing to do. Of course, this obviously limits a man's ability to realize the many benefits meditation has to offer. Anyone wanting to practice meditation, can do so at a very basic level or progressively higher levels of seriousness based on interest and commitment. At the basic level, meditation can be as simple as sitting in a comfortable position, trying to clear the mind by focusing on some pleasant thought, and breathing deeply for about 15 to 20 minutes. If you want to go to a more serious level, consider adding some or all of the following steps.

1. Find a quiet place where all distractions such as phones, doorbells, or other interruptions can be eliminated.
2. Wear very loose clothing.
3. Sit in a very relaxed but focused position (legs crossed with hands on knees is one common position).
4. Focus on one thing in the room and hum or say "your word" (mantra) over and over again to block out other thoughts.
5. Some people have had success with visualization techniques such as visualizing a thermometer dropping gradually or a clock going slower and slower. This can help to reduce your heart rate and blood pressure.
6. Sit straight, but relaxed.
7. Breathe rhythmically, even counting the time to breathe in and the time to breathe out.
8. When finished don't stand up immediately or move quickly. Allow some time for transition. Do some stretches and then move slowly from your sitting position.

There are many good books and videos for those interested in learning more about meditation.

Aromatherapy
Aromatherapy involves massaging essential oils into the skin, inhaling them, or using them in bath water. This may sound very

superficial, but aromatherapy is actually based on some very sound science. The oils extracted from flowers, leaves, seeds, roots, and stalks of aromatic plants and trees can have a very powerful and positive influence on our body. The oils rubbed or massaged into the skin reach our circulation system through tiny capillaries just below the surface of our skin and are in our bloodstream having their desired impact within 20 minutes. Inhaling the essence of these oils stimulates the limbic system in the brain, which controls our moods and emotions.

> The primary benefit of aromatherapy for smokers can be the relaxation of muscles, the soothing of air passageways, the reduction of stress, and relief from headaches.

These oils are created from a distillation process that produces a highly concentrated substance which means only small amounts are necessary. The primary benefits of aromatherapy for smokers can be the relaxation of muscles, the soothing of air passageways, the reduction of stress, and relief from headaches. This is especially helpful for people who are trying to reduce the number of cigarettes they smoke or quit altogether. Stress and headaches are two of the biggest complaints smokers have during this withdrawal period.

Here are some of the useful essential oils for smokers.

Essential Oil	Uses
Cajuput	Respiratory infections, coughs, sinus infections, colds, and sore throats
Cinnamon	Tones the circulatory and respiratory systems
Ginger	Strengthens the immune system
Lavender	Effective relief from headaches
Melissa	Relieves stress, migraines, and nervous asthma

Essential Oil	Uses
Myrrh	Helps with chronic respiratory conditions, mouth and throat infections
Peppermint	Effective on headaches and sinus congestion
Rose	Helpful with stress, anxiety, and depression
Sandalwood	Relieves throat infections and stress
Tea Tree	Helpful with respiratory infections, coughs, colds, and phlegm

Basic Use Guidelines for Aromatherapy
All oils should be diluted since they are too strong to be used directly on the skin.

Massage – A professional massage therapist is recommended. A few drops of the desired oil should be mixed with a teaspoon of a carrier oil, such as grapeseed or almond oil. A Swedish-type massage is usually recommended, as it will effectively work the oil into the skin.

Bathing – Add approximately five drops into the bath and soak long enough for good absorption (10-20 minutes).

Inhaling – Add three to four drops into a pan of hot water and cover your head with a towel while leaning over the pan for about five minutes of inhaling.

Aromatherapy Cautions
The following guidelines will help you enjoy the safe and successful use of aromatherapy.

1. Never swallow essential oils. Keep out of the reach of children.
2. Some oils are not suited for pregnant women. Check with your qualified health care professional.

3. People with severe asthma should consult their physician prior to the use of aromatherapy.
4. People with high blood pressure, diabetes, epilepsy, or skin disease should also check with their physician and an aromatherapist.
5. Never use essential oils near your eyes.
6. Be careful with citrus oils as some are toxic when exposed to sunlight.

Acupuncture and Acupressure
Acupuncture and acupressure are based on more than 3,000 years of experience in Chinese Medicine, and Western medicine is beginning to accept this ancient and powerful medical tool. The basic concept of acupuncture involves the existence of pathways or meridians in the body that carry our life force or energy. The Chinese call this qi (pronounced chi), while many Western practitioners equate it to the body's electrical system. If this energy or electricity flow is disturbed or blocked in any way, then illness can follow because the body is not in balance and not able to ward off illness and disease. There are 3,000 years of success behind this practice, and now there are several scientific studies supporting the benefits of acupuncture and acupressure. Thermographic pictures of injured animals show extreme inflammation that is greatly reduced within 20 minutes of an acupuncture treatment. No Western medicine or therapy can produce such quick and impressive results. Acupuncture, like any health protocol, has its strong suits, but it may not be the answer for everything.

Acupuncture is a licensed medical practice, and you should always ensure that your practitioner has the appropriate license. Acupuncturists are usually designated as Doctors of Oriental Medicine, and they will also incorporate the use of herbs in their treatment protocols. (More on herbs for smokers later in this chapter.) The D.O.M. (Doctor of Oriental Medicine) will use your medical history and a physical exam to determine your current state of health. The color of your skin and your tongue will be keys to this exam, as well as some touching of key parts of your body. By these methods they can tell how much impact smoking is having on your health. If you are toxic, they should be able to determine where the key blockages are and will try to reopen them with the placement of acupuncture needles. There is very little pain involved with the needles used in acupuncture. Obviously, if smoking is your concern, part of the doctor's treatment will be to improve energy flow to the lungs and the circulation system. Try a few treatments and see if you feel better. If not, perhaps acupuncture is not what you need at this time.

Herbal Medicine

Herbal medicine has been an integral part of the practice of medicine for over 5,000 years in every part of the world. Through trial and error, "doctors" have found the medicinal benefits of thousands of herbs and now they are finally being subjected to classic Western medical clinical tests. Not surprisingly, many of these ancient healing herbs are proving to have the precise healing properties that have been claimed through the millennia, and they are beginning to play an increasingly significant role in maintaining the health of many people. Popular herbs such as echinacea, aloe vera, garlic, and St. Johns Wort have evolved into the mainstream of public use and acceptance.

> Not surprisingly, many of these ancient healing herbs are proving to have the precise healing properties that have been claimed through the millennia, and they are beginning to play an increasingly significant role in maintaining the health of many people.

For smokers, there are many herbs and herbal formulas that have been shown to relieve certain common symptoms as well as boost overall health and improve specific body functions.

Symptom/condition	Herb
Wheezing	Bitter almond seed
Breathlessness	Red ginseng – also good for colds and poor circulation
Viral Infections	Echinacea, purpurea
Cough and colds	Garlic, hyssop, chamomile, seneca root, ginger, lemon balm
Allergies	Wild thyme, nettle, garlic, ginkgo
Sleep aid	Chamomile, hops, lemon balm, valerian
Stress	Valerian, chamomile, scullcap
Respiratory infections	Seneca root, skullcap, lomatium/osha formula
Bronchitis	Echinacea, garlic, mullein oil

Some Herbal Cautions

Echinacea – Patients with autoimmune conditions such as lupus, tuberculosis, multiple sclerosis, or AIDS should avoid echinacea.

Ginkgo (Ginkgo biloba) – Do not mix with anticoagulants (aspirin), Coumadin, Warfarin, Ticlid, or MAO inhibitors (Nardil and Parnate).

Goldenseal – Do not take with anticlotting drugs such as Coumadin or Heparin.

Valerian – Do not take valerian with anti-anxiety pills (Valium or Xanax), antidepressants (Elavil), anti-allergy drugs (Benadryl or Vistaril), or any herbal sedative.

St. John's Wort – Avoid using St. John's Wort with tetracycline, Prozac, Zoloft, MAO inhibitors (Nardil or Parnate), kava-kava, anticonvulsants, birth control medication, HIV medication, or any asthma medication.

Ginseng – Do not take with heart, blood pressure, or diabetes medication, MAO inhibitors, or caffeine.

Some herbs should be avoided by people with certain conditions, so you should seek more information about using the herbs listed. A good source to check possible contraindications (adverse reactions) is www.alternativedr.com. Consult articles appearing in *Herbs for Health* and other credible sources, and ask your health care provider for guidance. This list is for educational purposes only and not intended to be used as a self-medication guide.

Additional Guidelines for Using Herbal Remedies
• Buy herbs only from trusted and reputable sources such as health food stores, pharmacies, and doctors.
• Most herbs should not be taken on a continuous basis, because the body only "needs" them for special conditions. Always take a week or two off after a week or two of taking any herb.
• Read the label carefully to ensure the proper dosage is taken.
• Make sure your herbs are not too old. Check expiration dates, which apply to some herbs.
• If you are pregnant, seek the advice of your physician before taking any herb.

Homeopathy
Homeopathy is based on the principle that our bodies have the capability of healing themselves if they are encouraged to do so. When our immune system is overwhelmed by a particular illness it is necessary to stimulate that system to produce the appropriate antibodies to eliminate the substance or condition causing that illness. Homeopathy was founded on the belief that a very diluted version of the substance causing the illness can actually stimulate the body's immune system to produce a cure.

Homeopathy uses plants, minerals, and even some animal products as a base for its therapies. The homeopathic practitioner attempts to identify all of the underlying causes behind various symptoms, such as emotional and mental changes, as well as the more noticeable physical indicators. The overriding statement, which captures the essence of homeopathy, is "that which can cause disease can also cure it." Homeopathy can treat very acute symptoms safely and effectively with no side effects. It works with the immune system to create balance in the body's energy force. It improves resistance to infection, shortens recovery time, and often prevents more serious complications.

In homeopathy healing progresses from the more important organs to the less important ones, and symptoms usually disappear in the reverse order to their original appearance.

For smokers there are many potential uses for homeopathic remedies including the following symptoms or conditions.

- Effects of stress
- Depression
- Asthma
- Insomnia
- Headaches from withdrawal
- Coughs
- Nausea
- Suppressed immune system

Homeopathic remedies are often used independently from one another or other types of remedies such as herbs, vitamins, minerals, or other nutritional supplements. However, for specific conditions such as smoking cessation, detoxification, and immune system strengthening, it is possible to use homeopathy in conjunction with other remedies to produce a more effective formula.

This is the approach applied by Vaxa International in the development of the products used to support the smoking cessation protocol outlined in this book. As a registered Homeopathic Medicinal Company, Vaxa has many years of experience in combining homeopathic substances with other supplements to produce superior products. Two of the formulations developed for this program are featured in the appendices of this book.

Chiropractic and Osteopathy

Smokers might wonder how adjustments to the muscular skeletal system can have any impact on health issues related to smoking. Actually, there are many potential benefits to be realized by smokers who visit their chiropractor. Keeping the spine in proper alignment can ensure that the nerves serving the lungs are not blocked in any way. This ensures that the muscles controlling lung function are working properly and do not add to any problems the smoker may be having. Chiropractors and osteopaths can help keep people mobile and able to exercise. If you experience back pain or limb discomfort, this can reduce your ability to exercise, which can have a negative impact on your respiratory system.

The list of health issues potentially addressed by chiropractors and osteopaths include:

Breathing constraints – freeing the chest cavity of restrictions.
Headaches and migraines – releasing trapped nerves or relieving tension.
Neck, shoulder, and back pain – releasing tension and improving mobility.
Joint problems – improving mobility and reducing inflammation (any inflammation reduces the effectiveness of the immune system, which becomes overloaded and cannot help the smoker cope with other germs, toxins, or bacteria).
Irritable bowel syndrome – helps stimulate and free up the nerves serving the stomach and the digestive system (smokers need all of the nutrients they can get, which means they need their digestive system to work efficiently all of the time).
Bronchitis – can relieve stress on the respiratory system.

Many chiropractors and osteopaths are also knowledgeable about nutrition, supplements, and other alternative remedies. They can often help smokers, or anyone, to maintain good posture and muscular skeletal function, which in turn keeps other bodily functions working such as circulation, digestion, detoxification, and the endocrine system (i.e., hormones). Maintaining these and all body systems in top working order can help smokers greatly minimize the potentially negative impacts of smoking. As we will discuss later, by promoting good health on all of these "other" fronts, smokers may actually improve their ability to reduce their dependency on tobacco.

Hypnotherapy

Hypnosis is nothing more than a trance-like state of mind where someone can be very receptive to suggestions made by a hypnotherapist. This is important for someone who may be trying to replace old lifestyle habits with new ones in an attempt to become healthier. Many people have actually used hypnosis to assist in their efforts to quit smoking. It has been shown that 90% of people can be hypnotized by a professional hypnotherapist. Some people cannot be hypnotized because they are unwilling to relinquish enough control to someone else trying to influence their state of mind. Hypnosis is nothing more than a self-induced daydream with assistance from a trained professional.

> Successful hypnosis can reduce the craving for tobacco as well as increase the motivation to sustain new healthy living activities.

The key to successful hypnotherapy is achieving a high level of relaxation, which can be very useful in the treatment of things like stress, hypertension, migraines, and irritable bowel syndrome. It can also help people with lung related problems such as asthma, because it can help relax the key muscles of the throat and lungs. Many smokers also seem to use tobacco as a way to relieve stress, although we know it actually can have the reverse effect. Successful hypnosis can reduce the craving for tobacco as well as increase the motivation to sustain new healthy-living activities.

109

Hypnosis usually requires about six sessions, of one hour for each session, at which time the hypnotherapist may actually teach the patient to use self-hypnosis. The suggestions made by the practitioner usually involve some form of visualization where you picture either stopping something you don't want to do or doing something that you should do. It may be a less specific vision such as something calming or perhaps a suggestion to build your self-confidence. It is important to use a trained professional for this type of therapy and to remember that it is possible that repressed memories may be released as a result of your sessions. This should not be encouraged unless it is something you want to do and the practitioner is an experienced psychotherapist.

Biofeedback
Biofeedback is relatively new, compared to many other alternative therapies, having been developed in the 1930s. It shares similar principles with yoga, meditation, and hypnotherapy in that it emphasizes the use of techniques to gain more control over your body. By paying more attention to how your body is functioning and exercising self-control over things like breathing, heart rate, temperature, and blood pressure, we know that significant changes in the body are possible. These changes help the body to deal with stress, anxiety, depression, and other mental/emotional stimulation that can have a negative impact on a person's physiology. Smokers often experience these emotional/mental concerns and use smoking as one of their coping mechanisms. Biofeedback can help smokers get in touch with the negative reactions in their body and use a series of countermeasures to reverse and minimize the negative results of these reactions.

Actually, biofeedback can only work if it is used in conjunction with other techniques such as meditation, deep breathing, or even self-hypnosis. The biofeedback contribution often involves being hooked up to an electronic device capable of monitoring brain waves, heart rate, blood pressure, and skin temperature. As the various relaxation techniques are employed, it becomes possible to monitor the actual changes occurring in the body thus reinforcing the ability to learn which techniques are working best. When we experience this type of biofeedback, learning is greatly enhanced as the brain can imprint the success of the activity for future reference and repetition.

The measurable results of biofeedback experiments have included increasing the number of alpha brain waves (the relaxing ones), slowing of the heart rate, decreasing sweat gland activity, reducing skin temperature, and reducing blood pressure. As has been mentioned earlier, these changes lead to the production of anti-stress hormones, the relaxation of muscles, and the increased delivery of oxygen to our cells. For smokers, these are extremely useful changes that can at least partially offset some of the negative impacts of smoking.

One of the more recent developments in this field has been the computerization of biofeedback techniques by a company and technique named Heartmath. There are books on this research and a number of trained practitioners around the country who can provide individual or group sessions on the Heartmath technique. This is both a greatly simplified and a more technically sophisticated approach than previous biofeedback techniques.

Massage Therapy
There are many different types of massage, including Swedish, Shiatsu, Reiki, Tuina, and Thai. Each one has its benefits. Most Western techniques (Swedish) stress muscle massage, while most Eastern and Oriental techniques concentrate on the stimulation of acupressure points. Both types of massage can have benefits for smokers since one (Swedish) helps relax muscles and relieve stress, while the other (Oriental) helps improve energy flow in the body. However, there is another type of massage that may be even more helpful for smokers, and it is known as lymph massage. Lymph

glands are located throughout the body and serve as collection points for free radicals and other toxins that accumulate every day from the food, air, and liquids we consume. The lymph system collects these pollutants and then delivers them to the liver for processing in a controlled manner. If we become too toxic, the lymph glands will become clogged and swollen, which impedes their ability to function efficiently. Lymph massage is a technique for breaking up these clogged lymph glands and releasing these toxins for processing by the liver and the rest of our detoxification system. It is important to use a professional for any type of massage, especially the lymph type, because the release of too many toxins can overload the liver and possibly cause a negative reaction.

> There is another type of massage that may be even more helpful for smokers, and it is known as lymph massage.

Another benefit of lymph massage and other types of massage is the increase in killer cells (B cells and T cells), which are responsible for attacking germs and other invaders in our body. The lymph glands are one of the barracks where these killer cells wait to be called into action. They help to neutralize some toxins when they are brought to the lymph gland, but also go out on patrol to find toxins which haven't been brought in yet.

Many studies have been done to substantiate the benefits of massage including reduction of the stress hormone cortisol, increase in killer cells, reduction in muscle pain, release of tension, increased alpha brain waves, improved circulation, relief of anxiety and depression, improved alertness, and reduced fluid retention.

Many people practice massage on other family members, which is certainly better than no massage at all; however, there are definite advantages to using a professional or at least learning some of the more basic professional techniques and procedures. Some general suggestions include:

112

- Select a quiet place so your mind can relax.
- The surface should be firm and flat but also comfortable.
- The room should be warm to ensure the muscles are soft and subtle.
- Oils or creams are helpful because they make movement over the skin easier and can contain beneficial herbs or minerals.
- Give the massage in some kind of sequence (i.e., from top to bottom) and begin in a gentle way building up to any increased intensity, then ending in a more gentle way.
- Approximately 30 minutes is needed to gain most of the benefits, with 60 minutes being even better.

Cautions include seeking medical advice if you have a heart condition, varicose veins, acute back pain, blood clots, bronchitis, eczema, a fever, or are pregnant. Also, be careful not to massage any injured part of the body without prior approval from your physician (M.D., Chiropractor, Acupuncturist, or Osteopath).

Reflexology
Massaging the feet and hands with emphasis on specific pressure points was used by ancient Egyptian societies, as a part of Traditional Chinese Medicine, and by natives in North America. It was not identified as having potential benefits within Western medicine until 1913, when Dr. Fitzgerald found he could numb certain parts of the body by applying pressure to certain points on the patient's hands or feet. Using this technique, he was even able to operate on them, causing very little pain. Dr. Fitzgerald went on to establish 10 zones in the body, based on his experiments, and reflexology was reborn.

Reflexology seems to have been an early adaptation of the Oriental practice of acupressure and is based on the principle that calcium and uric acid deposits can build up at nerve endings, thus blocking the flow of the body's energy. By stimulating certain pressure points on the feet, these blockages can be freed. It is also believed that specific organs can be stimulated by putting pressure on certain points. This stimulation is felt to promote healing and has been used on such maladies as migraines, stress, back problems, irritable bowel syndrome, constipation, and premenstrual tension.

Smokers can benefit from reflexology because the reflexologist can stimulate circulation and lymphatic drainage with specific pressure points. By applying pressure on one specific reflex point, the solar plexus can be stimulated, thus encouraging the diaphragm and the lungs to relax. Other points can also stimulate the liver, the kidneys, the adrenal glands, and the pituitary gland.

The evidence to support the benefits of reflexology is still mostly anecdotal, but some studies have shown clinical proof of benefits. A good sign of the impact could be the aftermath of a treatment, since many people experience rashes, headaches, and frequent urination, which signals the body's desire to get rid of the toxins being released by the treatment. Smokers need to take every possible measure to detoxify their bodies so that their smoking habit does not cause their immune system to be overloaded. Reflexology may be a useful and desirable detoxification technique for some smokers.

Nutritional Therapy
Food is often overlooked as a way to help the body deal with certain health problems or conditions. Western medicine has tended to emphasize the treatment of illness with drugs or surgery as opposed to helping the body "heal itself." This symptom-based treatment approach is increasingly being replaced with a more holistic approach to healing as more and more clinical evidence is gathered to support the value of nutritional therapy and other natural therapies.

Smokers all realize that the mouth, throat, and lungs are the primary body parts impacted by their use of tobacco. After reading the previous chapters of this book, they will also realize that smoking can have a detrimental impact on almost every part of the body from skin and bones to circulation and the pancreas. In spite of a very long list of potential health concerns caused by smoking, there are many nutritional decisions that can minimize these impacts. The following recommendations are listed in somewhat of a priority order.

1. Eat a diet consisting of fresh fruits and vegetables, whole grains, brown rice, nuts, and oatmeal. This will provide the optimum level of nutrients your body needs to be healthy.

2. Avoid animal fat (meat, dairy, etc.). Especially avoid red meat and choose low-fat dairy if you must have dairy. Drink organic low fat milk if possible. Homogenization causes milk molecules to become extremely small and able to enter the bloodstream without being fully digested. Smoking tends to make your blood stickier because of the tar and nicotine. The combination of fat circulating in your blood and the increased stickiness leads to a quicker build-up of plaque in the arteries than is usually the case. Saturated fat and smoking creates a sticky fat stew in your arteries.

3. Include lots of garlic and onions in your diet because they contain quercitin, mustard oils, and disease-fighting nutrients. They also cause an enzyme to be produced that helps to release anti-inflammation chemicals in the body. (Tobacco has inflam-mation-inducing chemicals in it.)

4. Eat foods high in vitamin C such as red peppers, guavas, broccoli, oranges, spinach, and papayas. Each cigarette destroys from 25 to 50 mg of vitamin C, which is vitally important as an antioxidant and for over 300 other important functions such as the production of collagen. One of the reasons that many smokers have loose and wrinkled skin is the underproduction of collagen due to the lack of vitamin C in their bodies.

5. Eat plenty of orange-colored vegetables such as carrots and sweet potatoes, because they contain beta-carotene, which is a precurser to vitamin A. Vitamin A is one of the most important vitamins for the lungs and helps keep them functioning with a minimum of toxicity. Lung cancer patients are often treated with megadoses of vitamin A as beta-carotene.

6. Avoid caffeine, especially coffee, since people who drink coffee and smoke cigarettes have an increased risk of pancreatic cancer.

7. Eat frequent small meals if possible to improve digestion. A full stomach can put pressure on the lungs, which smokers do not need.

8. Include green drinks in your nutritional plan made from concentrated vegetable powder, barley grass, wheat grass, spirulina, blue green algae, or chlorella. These greens are high in vitamins A, B, and C, which are vitally important for everyone, especially smokers.

Special Nutritional Tip
Dr. John Gray, author of the famous book *Men Are From Mars, Women Are From Venus*, has written a new book on nutrition. In it he recommends the consumption of a special protein shake in the morning, which can increase the body's production of serotonin and dopamine. This is valuable for smokers who can reduce their addictive cravings by producing these positive hormones. It also helps promote a good night's sleep. During REM or deep sleep our body temperature increases thus inducing an accelerated state of detoxification which is very beneficial for anyone, but especially for smokers. The recipe for this shake appears in Chapter XII.

> During REM or deep sleep, our body temperature increases thus inducing an accelerated state of detoxification which is very beneficial for anyone, but especially for smokers.

XI. Managing Your Habit

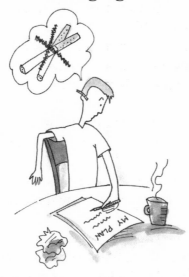

MARK TWAIN ONCE SAID, "QUITTING SMOKING ISN'T DIFFICULT, I've done it hundreds of times." People know how to quit; they just don't know how to stay that way. What many people have been able to do is cut back on the amount they smoke. This is easier because it retains some of the psychological and physical "benefits" people feel they get from smoking. The key is to be serious about your efforts to cut back, because if you aren't, the addictive nature of smoking can very quickly increase your need for nicotine in order to get the "normal" feeling that you crave.

Cutting back on the number of cigarettes smoked is highly advisable because there is a dramatic reduction in the negative impacts of smoking if you can get down to 10 cigarettes a day or less. Several studies have shown that the body seems to be able to tolerate this level of smoking fairly well, at least in most people. Add to that the benefits realized from the other changes recommended in this book, and you get very close to being the "healthy smoker" referred to in the title of this book. Changing your diet, exercising, taking supplements, and using various alternative health strategies could place the "10 cigarettes a day smoker" very easily in the top 10% of healthy people in the United States. Remember, over 63% of the population is overweight, and very few people exercise or eat very well. It's not really that difficult to be healthier than the average person these days.

Setting Goals is Crucial

We have all set goals at some time in our lives, and we know how important they are to achieving the things we really want in life. This is especially true when it comes to managing your smoking habit by cutting back on how much you smoke. Some people feel they are managing their habit if they smoke filtered cigarettes or cigarettes with less tar and nicotine. That may be true to some extent, but the best benefits come from the reduction of the actual number of cigarettes smoked. I can remember when my father cut back from two packs a day to four cigarettes a day. He did it over several months by setting specific targets for the number of cigarettes allowed each day. He even calculated when he would smoke each one and if he cheated during the day, he would just smoke half a cigarette at a time toward the end of the day so he wouldn't go over his limit. As I remember, his cut-back strategy became a little easier each week as he saw the success of his program. Finally, at four cigarettes per day, he felt he had achieved his goal and felt this small number was not causing him much harm. This was decades before any studies had confirmed that fact, but he knew how good he felt and by doing it slowly he was able to manage the weight gain problem many people complain about when they quit smoking "cold turkey." He maintained his same ideal weight of 173 pounds for the last 20 years of his life through good diet and daily exercise. He was a "healthy smoker."

Distractions and Substitutes

Many people report success in their cut-back strategies through the use of various distractions and substitutes for smoking. When it is your usual time to smoke, find something healthy to do instead.

Here are some ideas compiled from smokers who have successfully cut back on their smoking through distraction or substitution.

> Many people report success in their cut-back strategies through the use of various distractions and substitutes for smoking.

- **Eat a piece of fruit** – You can use this distraction one, two, or three times in a day. Eating more than that will cause you to eat too much sugar.
- **Eat nuts and seeds** – The B vitamins and nutrients in nuts and seeds will be welcomed by your body, and they are easy to carry with you all day. (Almonds, Brazil nuts, pecans, and walnuts are the best choices.)
- **Eat carrots, celery, etc.** – Vegetables are not as easy to carry around as fruit and nuts, but the vitamins and fiber you will get will be a blessing to your health.
- **Walk some stairs** – This will burn calories, clean out your lungs, and build muscle that will burn more calories. Remember to leave your cigarettes behind so you're not tempted to smoke.
- **Ride your bike** – The oxygen and exercise of biking will energize you, and the scenery is often helpful for stress reduction. Ride somewhere that is beautiful if you can.
- **Go for a walk** – Thirty minutes of walking is all you need in order to get major health benefits. Walk with someone and the time flies by as you catch up on each other's lives and reduce your stress through friendship and exercise.
- **Drink some water** – You won't always have a snack with you or the time to exercise. Good healthy bottled water helps flush out toxins from your body and keeps you hydrated.
- **Call someone you love or care for** – This is a perfect distraction because it takes your mind off the need to smoke and feeds your inner self.
- **Yoga or meditation** – Even deep breathing is good because the brain will produce positive hormones instead of the negative ones produced by smoking. Yoga and meditation are proven to reduce blood pressure and help create balance in your body.

Overcoming Barriers

In business, a forcefield analysis is often used to determine the forces for and against a certain plan or change in some part of the operation. Then managers and staff brainstorm some countermeasures to overcome the negative forces. This same technique can be used by smokers trying to develop a successful cut-back strategy. Simply list all of the forces for the cutback in cigarettes smoked each day, and the forces against, such as social event smoking, the habit of after dinner smoking, or the use of smoking as a procrastination tool to avoid making a decision. Then try to list all of the things you could do to overcome those barriers. You may be pleasantly surprised to learn that giving this much attention to your challenge pushes you toward taking more affirmative action. This is because you understand why you are smoking in certain situations and have decided to apply your intelligence and determination to overcome your barriers.

Journal Writing

Keeping a daily record of your efforts to reduce the number of cigarettes you smoke and improve your lifestyle habits is definitely a good idea. Journal writing has been proven as a successful tool in efforts to lose weight, stop smoking, stop alcohol consumption, exercise more, and a number of similar health improvement programs. Scientists contend that keeping a record helps strengthen the commitment to the desired change, allows for more accurate tracking of success or brief weakness, and increases the opportunity for positive self-talk. Knowing that you are going to record your actions seems to reinforce the pursuit of established goals. (An excellent journal-writing software program is available from www.lifejournal.com – Ruth Folit, developer.)

Journal writing can provide some other very specific benefits for people trying to manage their smoking habit by gradually cutting back. By keeping track of your various changes in nutrition, exercise, supplementation, and stress management, you can gauge how well you are meeting your goals in each of those areas. Specific changes can also be observed in your behavior patterns. For example, can you walk farther without getting out of breath? Do you have more energy, especially in the middle of the afternoon? Are you coughing less or getting fewer headaches if these were problems for you? By keeping a record of these positive aspects of your lifestyle changes, you can become your own cheerleader. Positive results can happen within a week or two, and isn't it better to be coping with such positive changes, rather than trying to cope with agonizing withdrawal symptoms? This is precisely why I feel so strongly that this strategy of becoming a healthy smoker is so much better than quitting cold turkey, at least for most people. Here are some of the categories that you may wish to monitor and a basic monitoring tool.

Symptom	Worse	Slightly Worse	Same	Slightly Better	Better
1. Irritability					
2. Insomnia					
3. Fatigue					
4. Dizziness					
5. Coughing					
6. Nasal Drip					
7. Dry Mouth and Throat					
8. Lack of Concentration					
9. Tightness in Chest					
10. Depression					
11. Constipation or Gas					
12. Hunger					
13. Craving for a Cigarette					
14. Headaches					

It is not absolutely necessary to use journal writing in order to keep track of changes in the above symptoms. You can decide to simply take this little test every month or so and use the results to both inspire you, and find areas where you may need to increase your efforts. For example, if you are experiencing headaches or depression, you may want to try to find a supplement to help reduce these symptoms. An excellent book for these emerging nutritional challenges is *Prescription for Nutritional Healing* by James Balch, M.D. and Phyllis Balch, C.N.C. Consulting a naturopathic physician is also a good idea.

Other Changes to Monitor

There are other emotional or behavioral changes you may also want to monitor because they can also help illustrate the positive results you are achieving with smoking reduction and lifestyle changes. Here is another chart you can use for these purposes.

Behavior Changes	Worse	Slightly Worse	Same	Slightly Better	Better
1. Mood Swings					
2. Sense of pride					
3. Relationships with others					
4. Self-esteem					
5. New friendships					
6. Peace of mind					
7. Procrastination					
8. Emotional stability					
9. Isolation					
10. Feelings of rejection					

Managing Other Dependencies

It is important during your efforts to cut back on smoking and change your lifestyle to watch for any desire to increase other harmful dependencies such as alcohol consumption or eating unhealthy foods. Cravings can sometimes jump from one area of dependency to another, especially if you are not monitoring your program very carefully.

Being proud of your progress in the area of smoking reduction does not give you the right to rationalize other bad habits or lifestyle choices. If you are on the watch for such problems, it is much easier to spot them before they become a serious problem. There are signs that you may be vulnerable to such changes or even a lapse in your cut-back strategy. Use the following scale to monitor your addictive behavior to see if any weaknesses are starting to occur as well as any progress you may be making.

> Cravings can sometimes jump from one area of dependency to another, especially if you are not monitoring your program carefully.

Addictive Pattern Changes	Worse	Slightly Worse	Same	Slightly Better	Better
1. Harbor feelings of suffering					
2. Lose count of allotted cigarettes					
3. Rationalize breaking your cut-back pattern					
4. Denying smoking's negative effects					
5. Smoking more when alone					
6. Cannot discuss smoking due to guilt					

123

Addictive Pattern Changes	Worse	Slightly Worse	Same	Slightly Better	Better
7. Avoid places that restrict smoking					
8. New cravings at normal smoking times					
9. Think more about smoking					
10. Tell lies about your smoking					

In order to assist you in this monitoring strategy, a workbook has been developed for use by anyone reading this *Healthy Smoker* book. A free copy of this workbook can be downloaded to your computer by going to www.thehealthysmoker.net.

Tracking physical symptoms, emotional patterns, and addictive behavior may seem like a time-consuming burden, but it really is a good test of your desire to make a positive change. If you are willing to make an honest and consistent effort to track your progress in this way, it is a true indication that you want to be successful.

Making a Plan

Managing a change as important and as difficult as cutting back on your smoking deserves a solid plan. Too many people fail in their efforts to quit or cut back because they take the challenge too lightly. They think they can just stop one day or cut back with no consequences. And they do this even though they have probably failed on many occasions, as did Mark Twain. However, as you can tell from the information presented in this book, the cards are stacked against such a naïve and unplanned approach.

> Too many people fail in their efforts to quit or cut back because they take the challenge too lightly.

124

Having a plan requires you to think about, and probably write down, some key information on the following topics.

1. Why did you start smoking in the first place?
2. Why do you continue to smoke?
3. In what situations do you usually smoke?
4. What makes it difficult for you to cut back or quit?
5. What was the reason you failed last time?
6. What illness symptoms do you already have?
7. Why do you think you won't get a serious disease?
8. What are the main reasons you don't want to become seriously ill?
9. Are you really exercising as much as you should?
10. Are you really eating as well as you should?
11. Why are you not taking the supplements recommended in this book?
12. Would stress reduction activities help you?

These questions should be answered in writing and lead to the development of a specific plan for cutting back. Divide your plan into stages and measure your progress at the end of each stage using the preceding evaluation tools. If you take this step to make a specific plan, you will greatly increase your chances of success. Go as slow or as fast as you think is reasonable for you. Generally, slower is better if you have smoked a long time and have many psychological and emotional challenges. Your body will need time to respond to the changes you are making. It is far better to take longer and succeed than to go faster and fail. (To assist in making your plan, a free workbook is available at www.thehealthysmoker.net.)

Rewards

For some reason we have become a society where rewards play a significant role in our lives, both at work and at home. Perhaps it stems from our early upbringing when parents tried to reinforce desirable behavior with some kind of reward. Whether it was good grades in school or finishing your dinner, there always seemed to be some tantalizing benefit waiting if we just "did the right thing." In too many cases, the rewards were even given for stopping something that we shouldn't have been doing. In other words, we were rewarded for just returning to normal behavior. If you stop crying we can go to the mall. If you clean up your room you can go out and play. And so it goes; we have nurtured this very strong need for rewards for positive behavior from a very early age.

This principle can be applied, in a constructive way, to the smoker who is trying to manage his or her habit and be carried out in many different ways. Smokers can reward themselves for meeting specific goals or even staying on their program. If you hit a target, treat yourself to dinner out or a mini-shopping spree. These rewards will register in your subconscious and begin to reinforce your commitment just as Pavlov proved with his little rats in the maze. As your accomplishments get bigger so can the rewards. By putting aside the money you are saving on cigarettes, you might get enough for that new DVD or that new piece of exercise equipment. How about a vacation when you reach a really big goal? Without getting into an extensive scientific explanation, suffice it to say that our brains produce chemicals that generate positive feelings in our bodies. These hormones can be released if we eat a food that we like, get a reward, or even smoke a cigarette. What you are actually doing with this reward system is replacing the "good feeling" that used to be generated by the cigarettes with another type of reward (a much healthier one). This will have a very significant impact on your ability to control your craving and better manage the addictive aspect of your smoking habit.

And finally, these rewards don't need to just come from you. Family members and friends should be encouraged to participate as well. Have you ever noticed that rubbing your own feet isn't quite as good as when someone else does it? The same is true with rewards, and this translates into the production of even more positive hormones in the brain and an even higher level of commitment to continue your program to its successful conclusion. Engage your significant other in this reward program because it is definitely in his or her best interest for you to be successful. Rewards are one of the best ways he or she can do this.

Final Words on Testing
Earlier in this chapter, we presented a number of tools to evaluate your progress in "managing your habit." All of these evaluation tools dealt with the soft side of evaluation such as symptoms, behavior changes, and addictive patterns. These are all good measuring sticks, but it is equally important to measure the actual changes taking place in your body. Here are a few tests described in Chapter IV, which you should consider using to gauge this physical impact of your program.

1. **Live blood cell analysis** – By looking at your blood cells under a microscope, you can determine if your blood is less sticky than it was before. This will require you to have a picture to compare what your blood looked like when you first started your cut back strategy. With all of the changes in diet, supplements, exercise, and stress management, you should see red blood cells that are better shaped, better colored, and not sticking to each other as much as they were before. This will be physical proof of your success and should be a strong motivation to continue. Wait least two months so the results will be more significant, and don't forget to get that reward for improvement.

2. **Oxygen levels** – One of your initial tests should have also determined the oxygen levels in your body. Chances are your level was in the 80s or low 90s when you started and should be moving to the mid- and even high 90s as you cut back on the number of cigarettes you are smoking. The test scale goes from 0 to 100 with 97 to 100 being an acceptable level of oxygen. Smoking reduces the body's ability to transport oxygen in our

blood cells to the other cells in our bodies, so this should definitely improve as you cut back, exercise, change your diet, and supplement.

3. **Antioxidant levels** – Another excellent test can measure the level of antioxidants in your body. Since smoking destroys vitamin C (25-50 milligrams for each cigarette), it stands to reason that cutting back should allow your body to preserve more of this valuable antioxidant. Add to this the increased consumption of fruits and vegetables, as well as the supplements recommended, and there should be an impressive improvement in the amount of antioxidants in your body. These tests are not always easy to find, but any good chiropractor or naturopath should be able to help you. In a pinch, call the vitamin maker Pharmenex because they have a program where health practitioners are able to measure the antioxidant levels of their patients. Their scale has a range of 0 to 80,000 with less than 20,000 considered poor. They use a blue light laser to measure the amount of antioxidants at the cellular level. There are also blood tests that can measure the antioxidants circulating in your blood.

4. **Symptoms Analysis** – Appendix VI provides a list of typical symptoms experienced when there is a deficiency of various nutrients in the body. As your Healthy Smoker Program is progressing, these symptoms should decline, which will provide another valuable indication of improved health.

In addition to getting a better antioxidant score, you should also notice that wounds heal faster, you get fewer colds, the flu doesn't last as long, and you get fewer infections. Keeping track of these benefits will give you tremendous confidence that your plan is working and that your entire immune system is functioning at a much higher level. This means you have also greatly reduced your risk of heart disease and cancer. This is the ultimate benefit for any smoker and should be considered the greatest reward of all.

XII. The Psychology of Quitting

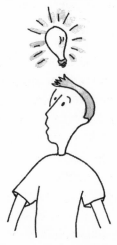

MOST SCIENTISTS AND INFORMED DOCTORS AGREE that most of smoking's power over the smoker is centered in the brain both biochemically and emotionally. The direct biochemical influence of smoking occurs when hormones called neuroregulators are produced in the brain as a result of smoking. Hormones such as adrenaline and dopamine allow smokers to actually control their feelings including becoming calmer or more excited. Short, quick puffs of a cigarette tend to arouse or excite brain function leading to an increased ability to concentrate. Longer puffs tend to create a more relaxed or calming effect, which is better for dealing with stress. Smokers can therefore control their moods with their cigarettes.

The less direct but equally powerful impact of smoking on the brain occurs when the smoker perceives the need for a cigarette based on a specific event or situation. The cigarette after dinner or after sex also produces a reaction in the brain as the memory of these pleasant experiences becomes attached to the habit of smoking just after they occur. The brain develops a pattern of connecting positive neurotransmitters on these occasions, and smoking becomes a reinforcing tool in this process. Our emotions can thus be further controlled with the habit of lighting up, which prolongs production of the feel-good hormones in our brain.

> Once smokers understand that there are much healthier ways to produce these same neuroregulators, then they begin to have viable options to their smoking habit.

Everyone knows how strong the addiction is to smoking, and this is confirmed by how difficult it is for most people to quit. However, understanding how this addiction occurs in the brain can help smokers to better appreciate the value of the cut-back and cessation strategies in this book. Once smokers understand that there are much healthier ways to produce these same neuroregulators, then they begin to have viable options to their smoking habit.

The Illusion of Normalcy

Smokers tend to think they feel better or normal only when they are smoking. Between cigarettes they are merely surviving until they can get their next fix. That is precisely why quitting is such an emotional challenge for so many smokers. They feel like they are giving something up, something they have come to depend on. Some smoking cessation programs are based almost solely on attacking this premise. They contend that quitting is not a sacrifice at all and, in fact, should be viewed as a new beginning of a healthier life. Of course, this is certainly part of the problem, but it belies the scientific evidence that smoking really does have a profound influence on the brain.

The argument used by some of the popular cessation programs is that smokers create most of the illusions of pleasure and need in their brains. They become friends with their cigarettes and feel that life would not be the same if they weren't able to share life's ups and downs with their "friends" as they have in the past. Some of these arguments have less credibility when you realize that the actual craving for a cigarette lasts three to five minutes for most smokers. If you can make it through that craving period you can actually survive without a cigarette for quite a long time. There is also the claim that 90% of nicotine leaves your body within three weeks of quitting, which is true and is one of the reasons why so many programs put so much emphasis on the first few days and the first few weeks. Then the question must be asked, why do so many people start smoking again within three months? Up to 70% of quitters make it past the first two months but can't seem to make it past three months. If it were just cravings and nicotine in the body, then this failure rate would not occur.

The Social Pressures
The answer to the 70% failure rate may be partially found in the socialization of smoking. Over the years smokers were drawn to "other smokers" as well as situations where "they would smoke." The social patterns of our life build a familiar and comfortable routine, which in turn gives us confidence and security. These are very strong psychological patterns that are sometimes less easy to change than the smoking itself. The visits outside to smoke with fellow workers or the bowling buddies who have shared many good times with you over the years are very strong bonds. When you see them smoking you are tempted to join them. That's when rationalization jumps in and says, *"Oh, just one cigarette won't do any harm."*

Rationalization: One of the Biggest Barriers
Our ability to rationalize may get us into more trouble than anything else we do. It can be traced back to many crimes as criminals rationalize their behavior as being justified because of all the wrongs they have endured. And so it is with smokers that they can call on rationalization to justify one more cigarette. They go even further to rationalize that they can quit any time they want to or that the diseases caused by smoking will happen to somebody else. This rationalization process is also impacted by the chemistry of the brain as the brain sends messages to defend its

> **Our ability to rationalize may get us into more trouble than anything else we do.**

source of adrenaline or dopamine. Cravings are the direct result of these biochemical influences, and rationalization is part of the long-term biochemical influence. This is precisely why it is so important to find some alternative hormone stimulators to satisfy the brain's needs. If this does not happen then eventually the brain will begin to send stronger and stronger messages demanding some source for these feel-good hormones.

Food as an Alternative
This brings us exactly to some of the problems quitters have with eating after they have stopped smoking. Certain foods, especially simple carbohydrates and sugars, also produce feel-good hormones in the brain. Sugar is especially powerful because tobacco is cured with corn or beet sugar, which means that smokers are inhaling large amounts of sugar every time they smoke. The combination of nicotine and sugar in the cigarettes has created a double dependency in the brain. After this source of neuroregulators has been removed, the brain naturally finds the perfect solution in the form of doughnuts, other refined carbohydrates, or even alcohol, which is basically sugar.

The alternative to these sugars and simple carbohydrates is obviously the more complex carbohydrates provided in whole grains, fruits, and vegetables. And as was mentioned earlier, positive hormones can also be produced by exercise, deep breathing, meditation, and the other natural therapies mentioned. Now it may be easier to understand why these lifestyle changes are so important to the would-be quitter. Without these changes the brain can continue to command the presence of cigarettes because the fix is so immediate. Nicotine gets into the bloodstream faster than almost any other substance, and it is the speed and effectiveness of this fix that the brain remembers so well.

> Nicotine gets into the bloodstream faster than almost any other substance, and it is the speed and effectiveness of this fix that the brain remembers so well.

The Rationalization Exchange Theory

The general influence of rationalization was discussed earlier. We now know that these urges in the form of cravings (short-term rationalization) and justification for continuing or starting smoking again (long-term rationalization) can be controlled to a great extent through changes in diet, exercise, and other natural therapies. There is another method of neutralizing this rationalization process, and that is to exchange one set of rationalizations for another.

In the case of existing smokers, they rationalize that smoking helps them cope with stress, avoid boredom, helps them to concentrate, allows them to function socially, and gives them something to do. It is also a perfect excuse to continue eating poorly, drinking alcohol, and not exercising because everybody knows you have to stop smoking before you should make any of these other changes. At least that is what many smokers do, because they have been told over and over again that smoking is their worst vice so they must stop that one first. We have already addressed this latter rationalization throughout this book by contending that smoking should be the last thing you change and not the first. At least this is probably true for most people. Once this overriding change in rationalization has taken place it should not be that difficult to exchange the other smoker's rationalizations for the quitter's rationalizations. Here is a sample exchange list.

Smoker's Rationalizations	Quitter's Rationalizations
• Stress relief	• Improves health – long term
• Boredom avoidance	• Increases energy
• Better concentration	• Saves money
• Social acceptance	• Improves self-respect
• Control of anger	• Better taste of food
• Keeps my weight down	• Improved sexual performance
• Helps control pain	• Fewer colds and infections
	• Fewer mood changes

By exchanging one set of rationalizations for another you can begin to move from the feeling of sacrifice to the feeling of liberation and rebirth. The changes you will make during this process will be among the most important in your life. You will have the confidence that you have regained control of your life and become an example to others around you who will be proud of your accomplishment. It takes more courage to change your life when a crisis is not present than to do so when directly faced with a crisis. Once the heart attack or cancer announcement has been made it is much easier to rationalize lifestyle changes because now the loss of life itself has become a real possibility. If, on the other hand, you rationalize that disease could happen to you, then you can begin the change process just described.

Competing Hormones
Our bodies are significantly influenced by the hormones we make each day, and smoking plays a big role in the production and suppression of hormones. We have mentioned two of these hormones, adrenaline and dopamine, but there are many others such as serotonin, cortisol, melatonin, and insulin, just to mention a few of the key ones. Each of these hormones plays an important role in our brains and our bodies, but some of them compete with one another and cause serious disruptions to our ability to maintain stable moods and a healthy chemical balance. Here are some examples:

- Adrenaline, which is triggered by stress or smoking, causes sugar to be dumped into our system for the energy needed to fight or run away (fight or flight reaction). Appetite is suppressed, blood thickens, cholesterol goes up, and our pulse increases. Adrenaline could save our lives, but if its production is stimulated too often it could be damaging to our bodies.
- Cortisol is produced when stress is very high or prolonged. Blood sugar increases as does the opening of fat cells to produce more energy. Inflammation declines initially and muscle tension increases in order to withstand physical challenges. Too much of this reaction is also harmful.

- Insulin is released to counteract excess sugar in the bloodstream and when fat cells open up. If sugar and fat aren't used through exercise then they are stored as fat in our cells. Cholesterol also goes up in these circumstances. This spiking of insulin is hard on the liver and the pancreas.
- Melatonin is the sleep hormone, and it is produced by the conversion of serotonin when sunlight entering the retina declines, thus sending a message to the pituitary gland. Darkness triggers this conversion of melatonin as serotonin is switched off, and deep sleep helps to restore body balance.
- Serotonin is the ultimate good guy in terms of hormones because it helps to lower stress, reduce cravings, reduce hunger, improve performance, and induce a positive mood state.

While most of the previously mentioned hormones are best kept at controlled levels, serotonin is the hormone you almost can't get too much of. It improves creativity, keeps you calm and self-assured, and generally promotes a sense of happiness. This is the very hormone you want to have more of in order to compensate for the stimulation usually received from smoking. If you have enough serotonin in your system your body will get a message from your hypothalamus that you have eaten enough after you have eaten. If you don't have enough serotonin this message isn't sent and you tend to overeat in search of more serotonin. Aggressive, angry, or depressed moods and headaches usually occur when people don't have enough serotonin in their system.

There are certain activities that stimulate the production of serotonin; these include:

- Therapeutic massage
- Exposure to sunlight
- Easy exercise such as biking, swimming, or walking
- Deep sleeping
- Positive thoughts or meditation
- Eating certain foods

The foods that help produce the most serotonin are the foods that contain high levels of tryptophan. These foods include the following:

• Almonds	• Cheddar cheese
• Chicken	• Kidney beans
• Salmon	• Scrambled eggs
• Cottage cheese	• Tuna
• Turkey	• Tofu
• Soy milk	• Cooked whole wheat spaghetti

There are also foods like ground beef and pork that contain high levels of tryptophan but they are not recommended because of their high fat content, the difficulty digesting them, and their contribution to certain types of cancer.

Eating some tryptophan-rich foods at as many meals as possible will certainly help any smoker who is cutting back or quitting altogether.

Some smokers have had great success with a special morning shake recommended by Dr. John Gray, who authored a new book entitled *The Mars and Venus Diet and Exercise Program*. In this book Dr. Gray recommends a shake with the following ingredients to produce high levels of serotonin. The formula is a little different for men and women.

Men	Ingredient	Women
30 g	Whey protein powder	20 g
4-6 oz	Oxygenated water	4-6 oz
2 tbsp	Almonds	2 tbsp
2 tbsp	Molasses	2 tbsp
1 w/skin	Apple	1 w/skin
1 tbsp	Flax seeds (ground)	2 tbsp

Men need a little more protein due to body size and women need a little more flax seed due to special hormone needs satisfied by the extra fat in flax seeds. Athletes boast of great energy surges when consuming this shake just after exercising. Others have raved about improved sleep. And ex-smokers say it keeps them calm, controls their cravings, and allows them to focus even better than when they smoked.

Subconscious Suggestions
We have already discussed how the brain is able to set up very strong suggestive messages connected with smoking and how these messages are reinforced biochemically in the brain. Earlier in this book we mentioned hypnotherapy as a natural therapy to help smokers in their efforts to cut back or quit smoking. Hypnosis is a very effective way to intercept these suggestive messages by replacing them with other more positive messages or messages against smoking. Everyone is not a good candidate for hypnosis, but for those who are, this has been shown to be one of the most useful tools in smoking cessation programs. Obviously we believe that hypnosis is even more powerful when it is used in combination with other strategies in this book.

The Psychology of Probability
The exact level of emotional and psychological challenge will be different for each smoker. This is the reason why some people can quit cold turkey, others have success with various cessation programs, and the majority of people do not succeed with any strategy. While our Healthy Smoker Program can increase the chances of success for most people it is not foolproof for everyone. Some people have too many barriers or challenges to overcome and may need even more help than the Healthy Smoker Program can provide. The following survey can help to determine the probability of success for most people.

Probability of Success Screening Test

Answer the following survey questions as honestly as possible in order to determine your probability of success in using the Healthy Smoker protocol in this book. Check the appropriate box.

1. Do you think about the future and feel that you have a lot to live for?

Points

Definitely Not	No	A Little	Sometimes	Definitely Yes
-1 point	0 points	+1 point	+3 points	+5 points

2. Have you successfully stopped smoking in the past for at least a three-month period?

Points

Never	Yes, less than 3 months	Yes, 3 months	Yes, more than 3 months
-1 point	+1 point	+3 points	+5 points

3. Do you have a fairly stable family life (very little stress or confusion)?

Points

Very Unstable	Unstable	Some Stability	Stable	Very Stable
-1 point	0 points	+1 point	+3 points	+5 points

4. Do you have a fairly stable work situation (low stress and good job security)?

Points

Very Unstable	Unstable	Some Stability	Stable	Very Stable
-1 point	0 points	+1 point	+3 points	+5 points

5. Do you take prescription medications or drink alcohol on a regular basis?

Points

5 or more per day	2-4 per day	1 per day	Occasional	Never
-1 point	0 points	+1 point	+3 points	+5 points

6. Do you consume caffeine on a regular basis (coffee, soft drinks, Red Bull, etc.)?

Points

5 or more per day	2-4 per day	1 per day	Occasional	Never
-1 point	0 points	+1 point	+3 points	+5 points

7. Do you now have or have you in the past had any serious acute or chronic illness (heart disease, cancer, diabetes)?

Points

More than 1	Only 1	Minor case	Never had any
-1 point	0 point	+3 points	+5 points

8. Are you able to avoid other smokers (in your family, at work or socially)?

Points

That's impossible	Not likely	Maybe	Doable	Very Doable
-1 point	0 points	+1 point	+3 points	+5 points

9. Do you feel that you have a fairly stable and healthy weight?

Points

10 lbs. under	20 lbs. over	10 lbs over	5 lbs. over	Ideal weight
-1 point	0 points	+1 point	+3 points	+5 points

10. Are you an organized person able to stay focused and on task most of the time?

Points

Never	A Little	Sometimes	Usually	Always
-1 point	0 points	+1 point	+3 points	+5 points

Each of these topics will have a bearing on how well people will be able to cope emotionally and psychologically with the challenge of becoming healthier and eventually stopping their smoking habit. After answering each question as honestly as possible, add up your score and see how challenging it will be for you to take advantage of the Healthy Smoker program.

Total Score _____

40 to 50 points = excellent chance of success
30 to 39 points = very good chance of success
20 to 29 points = a fair chance of success
 0 to 19 points = very low chance of success

If you scored low on this little survey it doesn't mean you cannot be successful. It simply means you will probably need a little more assistance than someone who scored higher. For example, you may need to consider one of the medications being used by some people to help them over their initial withdrawal and craving period. The best strategy would be to address the categories where you scored low first before trying to stop smoking. One small step at a time is exactly what is needed by some people, and this survey can help you determine which steps might be needed.

XIII. Cessation: Much Easier Now

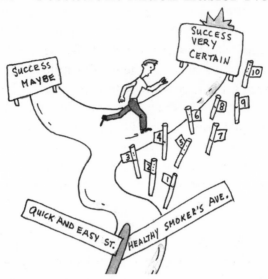

THAT FAMOUS QUOTE BY MARK TWAIN MAY BE FUNNY at first reading but it turns pathetic when you think about it. *"Quitting smoking isn't difficult; I've done it hundreds of times."* Yes, Mark, we get your point, but even a famous humorist like yourself would have to admit that these words say as much about the addictive nature of this unhealthy habit as they do about the lack of personal strength and judgment which accompanies it. Smoking may have even been fashionable in Mark Twain's time and stayed fairly unchallenged well into the 1950s and 1960s. However, it doesn't resonate very well in this century based on all of the knowledge we have about the health problems associated with smoking.

Phillip Morris was the biggest advertiser in the *Journal of the American Medical Association* in the 1940s, and at the AMA convention in 1947 Camel cigarettes had an exhibit that featured a banner proclaiming, "More Doctors Smoke Camels Than Any Other Cigarette." Only in the 1950s did this outrageous connection start to diminish as more and more evidence linked smoking to lung cancer. However, the AMA Retirement Fund still held tobacco stock well in the millions of dollars in the early 1980s.

Is it any surprise then that most doctors don't have very much to offer when it comes to advising their patients about how to quit smoking? Having received virtually no training about nutrition in medical school, and thinking that most disease is caused by outside forces that must be cut out, chemically killed, or radiated, most doctors haven't a clue about how to help smokers become healthier so they can quit smoking. Their simple, and not very helpful, advice is to just quit. If it were that easy to do even the rather intelligent Mark Twain would have been able to do it. (Note: The AMA has recently added a smoking cessation program to its website due to the commitment and research of a few of its more progressive members.)

Smokers Want to Quit

In various surveys it has been established that over 90% of people who smoke would like to quit. A majority of smokers have tried to quit but found it too difficult because of the strong addiction involved (i.e., as much or more addictive than cocaine or heroin, according to some doctors). The relapse rate for quitters is very high with 70% starting again within three months, because about 80% of these would-be quitters will experience serious withdrawal symptoms. These symptoms include irritability, sleep disturbances, anxiety, confusion, impatience, poor circulation, restlessness, headache, and gastrointestinal disturbances.

In spite of these serious withdrawal symptoms, some people are able to persevere each year and successfully kick the habit. Most are not successful and soon succumb to the craving for a cigarette that will end all of those nasty withdrawal symptoms. These withdrawal symptoms are due to the cellular dependence that has been created as cells in the brain want the endorphins, dopamine, beta-endorphins, and other hormones that are induced by nicotine. The whole body can get in on this stimulation that can run the gamut from calm to arousal. Smokers can even control which type of feeling they get by how much they inhale and how quickly they inhale. The physical and emotional dependency is simply too much for most people to deny as 60 trillion cells await the next fix with eager anticipation.

Why It's Easier to Quit Now
If a smoker has followed the health improvement guidelines contained in this book, it should be much easier to quit than it would have been if these guidelines had not been followed. Cellular dependency should decline as accumulated toxic material is removed from the body and new cells are given a chance to be healthier due to all of the nutrients and oxygen circulating in the body. With a large dose of antioxidants circulating in the bloodstream waiting for the free radicals created by smoking, it becomes more difficult for smoking to damage cells and work their addictive magic. Curcumin is on guard protecting cells in the lungs, vitamin C is protecting cells in the arteries and elsewhere, vitamin E is on guard in the heart, and other nutrients help protect other body organs, systems, and functions. The body and the brain now have an army of nutritional defenders all helping to greatly minimize the negative effects of smoking.

With this cleansing, and the diminished negative impact of smoking, the opportunity to cut back on the number of cigarettes smoked each day could not be better. Gradually, over several weeks, a good cut-back strategy can work miracles with the help of the various lifestyle changes that have been made. Once the daily cigarette count has been reduced to less than 10, it is time to think seriously about quitting. Many studies have shown that the addictive nature of smoking is very low at 10 cigarettes a day or less. Even though this is true, it may still be difficult to finally quit. This is precisely when one of the many quitting strategies can be put to very good use. There are several to choose from, and most will work very well now that the level of cellular dependence has been significantly reduced.

The Most Popular Cessation Programs
Although there are many programs to help people quit smoking, there are some generic rules or guidelines that seem to apply regardless of which one you choose.

1. **Be sure you are ready** – Unless you are really ready to quit there is little chance that you will be able to do so. There are times when your stress levels, or other reasons for dependency, may not be appropriate to take this major step. Also, you must be sure that you can do it. Self-doubt is never a very good companion when you start a journey this difficult.

2. **Understand it is a process** – Quitting is usually not a one-time event that is over as soon as you put down your last cigarette. It is a process that may take weeks or months to complete, and you need to be prepared for this fact.

3. **General tips** – For those of you not participating in a formal (commercial) cessation program, there are a number of helpful tips that can help you along the way.
   • Find a friend to quit with you.
   • Throw away all ashtrays and smoking apparatus (lighters, etc.).
   • Keep your best quit-smoking book with you as a reminder.
   • Get your teeth cleaned the day you quit and vow to keep them clean from that day on.
   • Avoid alcohol, especially if it reminds you of smoking.
   • Avoid caffeine if it reminds you of smoking and also because it is not very good for you.
   • Carry healthy snacks with you at all times to satisfy oral cravings.
   • Write the reasons for quitting on 3x5 cards and carry them with you as a reminder.
   • Stay relaxed by getting a massage, taking a warm shower or bath, or practicing deep breathing.

- Get your house professionally cleaned and painted to get rid of smoke residue and smell. Vow not to soil your house or apartment again.
- Get all of your clothes cleaned to rid them of the smell of tobacco.
- Ask your friends and family to actively support you in your efforts to quit.
- Have your car cleaned to remove any tobacco smell.
- Help someone else who is trying to quit.
- Adopt a new hobby or craft that keeps your hands busy.
- Avoid social gatherings during the first few weeks if they will present opportunities to smoke.
- Keep a daily journal of your triumphs when smoking was avoided as well as a record of your improved health and well-being.
- Give yourself small rewards or treats for making it through specific situations or reaching target dates.
- Allow your pride and self-esteem to grow.
- Start thinking about your next self-improvement project because now you have proven how strong you are.
- Calculate the money you have saved, and do something nice for yourself or, better yet, for someone else.

Join Nicotine Anonymous
This is a spiritual program modeled on the Alcoholics Anonymous program, and it follows 12 steps:

1. We are going to know a new freedom and a new happiness.
2. We will not regret the past nor wish to shut the door on it.
3. We will comprehend the word serenity.
4. We will know peace.
5. No matter how far down the scale we have gone, we will see how our experience can benefit others.
6. That feeling of uselessness and self-pity will disappear.
7. We will lose interest in selfish things and gain interest in others.

8. Self-seeking will slip away.
9. Our whole attitude and outlook on life will change.
10. Fear of people and of economic insecurity will leave us.
11. We will intuitively know how to handle situations that used to baffle us.
12. We will suddenly realize that God is doing for us what we could not do for ourselves.

Try the Patch
There are various patches of different strengths, which can release drugs into the body that reduce the physical cravings for nicotine. One of these uses clonidine, which has some side effects such as drowsiness and dry mouth. Users of this type of patch should avoid alcoholic beverages and should have their blood pressure and heart rate monitored weekly. You should stop using the patch if the skin by the patch becomes irritated, your blood pressure or heart rate changes, you become drowsy or light-headed, or you experience any unusual reactions.

The One Shot Approach
There are clinics popping up in communities across the country that offer a one-injection solution to smoking cessation. For a fee ranging from $350 to $650, these clinics guarantee that you will be able to stop smoking as a result of this injection. One such clinic is called Lifeline Stop, and locations can be identified by going to the Internet and typing in Lifeline Stop. The details as to side effects and the actual success of this approach are not readily available.

Hypnosis
Many doctors and other health practitioners have proclaimed the effectiveness of hypnosis in helping people to stop smoking. I have known people who were successful using this approach, and I have known some who were not successful. Hypnotic suggestion is a very strong subconscious tool, but in some people it is not strong enough to overcome the addictive or social powers of smoking. It

is difficult to pre-screen those who might be successful at hypnosis other than to say that strong-willed people with long-term addictions are not the best candidates.

The Juice Fast

Dr. James Balch reports that many people have stopped smoking by going on a juice fast. Consuming fresh juices and distilled water can apparently remove nicotine from the body very quickly and has achieved the desired results in just five days. Fasting is a very sensitive technique that should be closely monitored by a qualified holistic health practitioner. A naturopath or holistic medical doctor would be preferred since they understand the body and how it works biochemically.

Homeopathic Assistance

Controlling withdrawal symptoms is often the biggest problem faced by quitters. Natra-Bio Homeopathic is a company that markets a product named Smoking Withdrawal that has been proven to help manage withdrawal symptoms.

Buproprion (Zyban)

This is actually an antidepressant that acts on the brain in much the same way nicotine does. It may also assist in controlling weight gain after quitting, which is a common problem among many ex-smokers. The caution is to make sure you don't simply trade in one addiction for another.

Other Types of Products

There are many other products available to assist smokers who would like to quit smoking, including nicotine substitute chewing gums, nasal sprays, and inhalers. As with any of the above techniques, it is advisable to verify safety and effectiveness before trying them.

Other Sources of Assistance

There are numerous organizations, help lines, and websites designed to help people quit smoking.

1. *No If's, And's, or Butts, The Smokers Guide to Quitting* by Harlan M. Krumholz and Robert H. Phillips. A comprehensive guide with numerous strategies for quitting.
2. *Recovery from Smoking* by Elizabeth Hanson Hoffman, Ph.D. and Christopher Douglas Hoffman, L.S.W. Includes a 12-step program that is decidedly aimed at those with a more spiritual approach to life.
3. Nicotine Anonymous World Services – 2118 Greenwich Street, San Francisco, CA 94123 – Phone: 415-922-8575.
4. The American Lung Association – 1740 Broadway, New York, NY, 10019. They publish a book entitled *Freedom From Smoking for You and Your Family.*
5. The American Cancer Society – 4 West 35th Street, New York, NY 10001. Their Fresh Start program features four one-hour sessions over a two-week period. They also produce a free handbook called *I Quit Kit.*
6. U.S. Department of Health and Human Services – 800-784-8669 or www.smokefree.gov.
7. Smokers Anonymous – P. O. Box 25335, West Los Angeles, CA. 90025. They provide information on support groups for those who want to be quitters.
8. www.TheHealthySmoker.net

The Benefits of Quitting

The benefits of not smoking obviously bear a very close resemblance to the negative impacts of smoking mentioned in Chapter III. However, repeating the short- and long-term benefits of quitting is appropriate as you look forward to the successes achievable by following the guidelines in this book.

Short-term Benefits
1. Carbon monoxide in your blood declines within eight hours of quitting.
2. Food will taste and smell much better.
3. Respiratory function will improve, including less coughing and reduced production of phlegm.
4. Sexual function will improve, especially for males.
5. Increased stamina and vigor will occur as a result of increased circulation of oxygen to the cells.
6. Self-image and self-esteem should improve as you feel the pride of accomplishments as well as the freedom from your previous addiction.
7. Blood pressure should decline as well as heart rate and body temperature.
8. Your breath will be fresher, and you will no longer smell like a walking ashtray.
9. You will have fewer colds and infections.
10. You will save money.
11. You will no longer feel like a social outcast.
12. If you have a disease, such as heart disease, you will notice reduced symptoms, such as reduced chest pain, almost immediately.

Long-term Benefits
1. The risk of premature death will be greatly reduced.
2. The risk of heart attack will decline after just one year, and after seven years your risk will be similar to someone who has never smoked.
3. The risk of lung cancer will be 60% lower after six years and will be the same as a nonsmoker after 15 years.
4. The risk of cancer of the larynx will continuously decline until, after 10 years, it will be equal to that of a nonsmoker.
5. The risk of birthing problems such as stillborn babies or low-birth-weight babies is reduced when a woman quits smoking.
6. The ability of your body to heal improves. Better oxygen and nutrient circulation is the key to better healing.

7. Improved performance in physical activities such as sports, dancing, and other activities should be possible.

8. The risk of cancers such as bladder cancer or cancer of the mouth is greatly reduced to the level of nonsmokers in seven to ten years.

9. Headaches and mood swings will be greatly reduced for many people after they quit smoking.

10. Asthma and allergy sufferers should realize substantial relief from their symptoms. If the diet and supplement programs recommended are continued, many people should be able to become completely symptom-free in just a few years.

11. The risk of glaucoma, cataracts, macular degeneration, and other diseases of the eyes will be greatly reduced.

12. Brain function should improve with the possible reduction of diseases such as tinnitus (ringing in the ears), Alzheimer's, and Parkinson's disease.

13. Diabetics should realize a significant reduction in symptoms and complications. In many cases those suffering from Type II diabetes who follow the recommended diet and supplement program can actually get off their medications by adding specific supplements that help balance blood sugar (i.e., chromium picolinate, plant sterols and sterolins, reduced L-glutathione, vanadium, alpha lipoic acid, and L-carnitine).

14. Women can experience an increase in fertility, and men can increase sperm count, which means couples can increase their chances of achieving pregnancy and having a healthy baby.

15. Stress levels should be greatly reduced, especially if the nutritional, supplementation, and deep breathing or meditation changes are continued.

16. The immune system should be significantly enhanced which translates into a vastly improved ability to ward off every type of disease and illness that might be encountered.

XIV. The Ideal Healthy Smoker Protocol

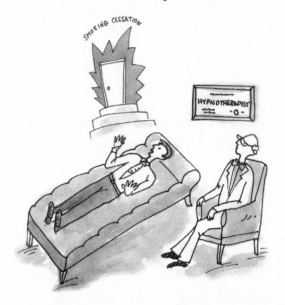

THERE HAVE BEEN MANY SUGGESTIONS OFFERED in this book about how smokers can become healthier in order to make it easier to quit smoking. The list of these recommendations should be thought of as a shopping list from which smokers can select the things they think will work best for them. There are some Healthy Smoker elements that are more important than others and therefore are more strongly recommended to be an integral part of every smoking cut-back and cessation program. To make it a little easier to consider all of these recommendations, this chapter will feature an ideal Healthy Smoker Program, which has been determined to be the easiest and most highly effective combination of the various elements in this book.

Step I – Set Some Goals – Based on the information in Chapters I and II, what are some of the reasons why you want to get serious about becoming healthier so you can eventually quit smoking?

1. What are the three things you think smoking does for you that are going to be difficult to replace with healthy alternatives?

2. What are the three highest priority lifestyle improvements you are interested in achieving such as more energy, better sleep, better sex life, etc.? What improvements are you seeking in your quality of life?

3. What are the three most important health issues you wish to address by becoming healthier? Which illnesses or diseases concern you the most based on your family history, your current health status, or just those health issues of most concern to you?

Write these statements on a sheet of paper and let it be the first page in a binder you are going to start which will hold all of the documentation that is a part of this program. You should know by now that the quick and easy approaches to smoking cessation don't work for most people, and everyone is just a little bit different in terms of their situation. This binder will be the smoking cessation program that you designed, not someone else.

Step II – Get Some Tests – There are several different tests mentioned in this book and they all can provide valuable information on your current health. However, very few smokers will have the time, the money, or the interest in getting all of these tests. Also, many of these tests may not be covered by conventional insurance policies. Therefore, it may be better to stick with a few tests that are easier and likely to be covered by insurance.

1. A comprehensive blood test can include many health risk factors, but often some key ones are left out. Ask your doctor to include a test for C-reactive protein, which measures the presence of inflammation in the body. Also, ask the doctor to get measurements of toxins in your blood as well as antioxidants or vitamins. This will not be as good as getting measurements at the cellular level such as those available from hair analysis or blue light laser readings, but they will still give you some information on the toxins and antioxidants circulating in your blood. Also, this type of test is usually covered by insurance.

2. Testing your acid/alkaline balance is very easy, because you can buy the test strips at any drugstore and test yourself in the morning. This will let you know how acidic your body is and thus how vulnerable you are to disease.

3. Most doctor checkups include a test for blood pressure, which is crucial because smoking has such a negative impact on circulation.

4. Most doctors should also be able to do a lung capacity test which will provide an excellent assessment of how much harm your habit has already done to your lungs.

These basic tests will provide some benchmarks against which you can measure the success of your Healthy Smoker Program. Of course the best test will be how much better you feel. If you want to use the comprehensive five-second test used by acupuncture physicians, then just stick out your tongue. If it has a white coating on it your health is not what is should be. When you are really healthy your tongue should be a beautiful pink color on the total top surface. When you have this color on your tongue you will be a very healthy person. Keep the results of these tests in your binder.

Step III – Detoxification – Toxins come from many sources, but smoking is the most toxic source for most people who smoke. By cutting back you will be eliminating a large percentage of your current toxic burden. There are other sources of toxins, and anyone would be wise to take the avoidance steps listed in this book. However, in our ideal program these are the priority detoxification steps to take.

1. Add the cleansing foods mentioned in Chapter V to your regular diet.
   - Spinach
   - Cabbage
   - Cucumbers
   - Watermelon
   - Beets
   - Celery
   - Fish
   - Pumpkin

• Carrots	• Raw fruits	• Chicken	• Guavas
• Asparagus	• Olive oil	• Watercress	• Soy foods
• Parsnips	• Brussels sprouts	• Figs	• Garlic

2. Order the detoxification formula from Vaxa International and take it for the recommended four-week period. Don't forget to purchase the cell rebuilding support product also, because your cells will need to be rebuilt after years of abuse.

3. Find a way to sweat every day either by walking as fast as you can without straining yourself or going for a steam bath or a sauna. The skin is the second most important detoxification organ after the liver.

4. Buy some detox tea and drink it in the evening after dinner. it will help with the overall detoxification effort and is very easy to do.

Step IV – Digestion – Good digestion is essential to becoming healthier and Chapter VI has many suggestions for improving the digestion process. There are several small steps that should definitely be an integral part of every Healthy Smoker Program.

1. Buy whole natural foods and avoid processed foods as much as possible. Include plenty of fiber, which includes whole grains, whole grain cereals, raw fruits, raw vegetables, and whole grain rice.

2. Do not overcook vegetables as heat destroys enzymes that are important to digestion. Eat a salad to begin dinner in order to activate enzymes, and if you are over 40 years of age consider using digestive enzymes before meals, because natural enzyme production declines with age.

3. Chew your food a lot or it won't be properly digested, which means you will not get all of the nutrients in the food.

4. Eat five or six small meals throughout the day if possible. If this is not feasible, eat three medium-sized meals with healthy snacks in between. It is extremely difficult to digest large meals, and your organs are designed for a steady flow of foods with short times in between.

5. Eat yogurt regularly and consider taking supplemental acidophillus periodically to keep the bacteria in your intestines properly balanced. Good digestion depends on this.

Step V – Nutrition – Some initial guidelines have already been established in the previous steps dealing with digestion and detoxification. However, there are a few additional suggestions to round out the ideal eating program for healthy smokers.

1. Avoid junk food that has very little nutritional value.

2. Processed foods are almost as bad. That means almost anything that comes in a box, a can, or a jar.

3. Avoid saturated fats such as red meat, dairy products (except fat-free) and anything fried.

4. Try to steer clear of stimulants such as alcohol, coffee, and most teas. (Green tea and detox teas are the exception.)

5. Don't forget to include some strawberries, grapes, and cherries, which are great for neutralizing the hydrocarbons found in cigarettes.

6. Drink plenty of water (filtered, spring, or distilled) in order to keep cells hydrated and help with the cleansing process.

7. Get your calcium from dark green vegetables, sardines, yogurt, or a supplement (not Tums).

Step VI – Supplementation – There are literally dozens of vitamins, minerals, herbs, and homeopathic remedies that are very important for smokers, and they are presented in Chapter VIII of this book. It is not reasonable to expect most people to consume so many separate supplements throughout the day, so a special combination supplement has been developed.

1. Order the sustaining supplement formula from Vaxa International and take it as directed on the label.

2. If you have specific vitamin deficiencies determined by the evaluation tool in Appendix VI, a test you have taken, or an assessment by a health practitioner, then you may need to take an extra supplement to meet these needs.

Step VII – Exercise – There are several possibilities in this book for a beginning exercise program or even more advanced activities for smokers who are already active. However, most smokers are not very active, so the suggestions in this ideal program are aimed at their needs.

1. Get your doctor's okay for whatever you decide to do.

2. Do something aerobic like walking fast or biking. Make your lungs work and increase your pace and/or time you do this exercise. (Every day if possible.)

3. Do something to build strength such as push-ups or some basic arm exercises. (Every day if possible.)

4. Do something for flexibility like yoga or tai chi.

These are just basic suggestions. If you prefer swimming, dancing, or some other activity, that is great. Just try to do something on a regular basis that uses as many muscles as possible and gets your lungs working. Believe it or not, this will be the one thing in your program that makes you feel much better very quickly. Nothing else will give you as positive a result as a little exercise.

Step VIII – Natural Therapies – There are several natural therapies that can be used by smokers to address a variety of health concerns or prevention strategies. These therapies are usually selected on the basis of very individualized needs and circumstances. However, there are a few natural therapies that are easy to do and are generally considered to be good for anyone on his or her way to being a healthy smoker.

1. Massage therapy is extremely beneficial because it is easy and is beneficial in so many ways. It helps reduce stress, improves circulation, and assists the detoxification process, just to mention a few of the more obvious benefits.

2. Aromatherapy is also relatively easy to utilize. Follow the directions in Chapter X for relief from some of the common symptoms experienced during withdrawal from cigarettes.

3. Deep breathing can be done anywhere and almost anytime with immediate benefits such as stress reduction and increased oxygen to the brain as well as to other cells throughout the body.

Natural therapies such as hypnotherapy and acupuncture are also very effective in the control of cravings and the emotional pressures to continue smoking. However, these therapies require confidence in the practitioners as well as the theory behind the therapy. This makes these, and the other natural therapies covered in Chapter X, very personal choices.

Step IX – Managing Your Habit – In the first step of this ideal Healthy Smoker Program you made a basic plan with some goals to help motivate you. In order to monitor your true progress during this program it will be very helpful to have a few monitoring tools. These tools will allow you to keep track of your progress on a regular basis and remind you where you began your journey. Chapter XI has a number of monitoring and motivational tools you should seriously consider.

1. A specific cut-back strategy should be included such as one less cigarette each week. You should also consider which cigarettes would be the best to eliminate first.

2. A substitute strategy should be included. What will you do instead of that cigarette – go for a walk, eat some fruit, or write in your journal? It should be something helpful and/or healthful.

3. Start a daily journal even if it is only a few lines each day. Journals not only allow for an outlet for your feelings, they also serve as a reminder of the reasons you are on this mission.

4. Fill out the Symptom Rating Scale, the Behavior Rating Scale, and the Addictive Patterns Rating Scale (*See* Chapter XI) on a monthly or a bi-weekly basis because this will help to hold you more accountable and be a real motivation to succeed.

5. Give yourself some rewards as you go forward in order to re-inforce your new positive behavior. Chapter XI has some good reward ideas.

Step X – Cessation – There are a number of suggestions about how to take that final step to quit smoking. However, it is hoped that most of them will not be necessary. If you have stayed with the Healthy Smoker Program then things like the patch or the shot should not be needed. This is especially true if you have been able to cut back to fewer than 10 cigarettes per day. Some very basic cessation steps should be the only things you need to do.

1. Pick a date and be determined to stick by your decision.

2. Get everything cleaned from your teeth to your car and your house.

3. Find someone to quit with you, but only someone who will also have a high probability of success (i.e., someone who has also gone through the Healthy Smoker Program).

4. Review your progress because now that your health is much better, you never want to jeopardize it again.

5. Consider hypnosis because now would be the perfect time to put smoking out of your mind. Your physical cravings will be much less, but your emotional and psychological cravings might still be there. Hypnosis can be a very useful tool to control these mental and emotional aspects of your former habit. (A hypnosis/meditation CD is available. To order this CD, go to www.TheHealthySmoker.net.)

If you have stayed very close to this ideal program, your chances of success have likely increased by as much as 90%, because you have addressed smoking cessation in the most comprehensive manner ever devised. Congratulations for your hard work and commitment.

The Workbook
To make it as easy as possible to follow this Ideal Healthy Smoker protocol, a workbook has been developed to guide your cut-back and cessation efforts. The workbook contains every assessment tool and checklist recommended in this book along with worksheets for making your plan and monitoring your success. The workbook can be downloaded at no charge by going to www.TheHealthySmoker.net. You will also find useful information for supporting your program such as recommended supplements (at discounted prices) and some specially designed products to make your efforts easier and more successful.

Appendix I

Essential Healthy Smoker Supplements
These four products are considered essential for everyone following The Healthy Smoker protocol.

Craving Control Spray – This homeopathic formula helps control the cravings smokers may experience as they cut back on the number of cigarettes they smoke. To be used as required within any limitations on the label. (To be used during all 3 months.)

Detoxification Formula – The vitamins and herbs contained in this formula support the body's natural detoxification process at the cellular level, in the liver, and throughout the body. (Used in month #1.)

Cell Rebuilding Formula – This vitamin and herbal formula helps provide the nutrients that may have been destroyed or impeded by smoking. This can help promote the cellular health necessary for the proper functioning of all organs and systems. (Used in month #2.)

Sustaining Multiple Vitamin – This special formulation of vitamins, minerals and amino acids complements a healthy diet to ensure the optimum level of nutrients are available to sustain nonsmokers on an ongoing basis. (Used in month #3 of the program and continuously thereafter.

Note: These four essential products are sold as a package with the price set at printing of $139.00. Prices subject to change due to the cost of ingredients. (1-877-476-6653)

Complementary Healthy Smoker Supplements
These products are provided to support the special needs of some smokers during their cutback and cessation efforts.

Buffer-pH – This product can help smokers to achieve a proper pH balance, which is crucial in helping to slowly dissolve calcified plaque and release trapped acidic residues.

Lung Formula – Promotes the body's natural process of respiration while providing nutritional support for the lungs.

Nite-Rest – Helps the body naturally to reduce restlessness, anxiety, nervous exhaustion, and insomnia.

Extress – Provides the body with the specific dietary require-ments that aid in its natural processes during periods of stress, tension, and anxiety.

Omegacin + – Contains 38 bioavailable fatty acids including Omega 3-6-9 necessary for cellular membrane integrity and optimal cardiovascular and central nervous system functioning.

Note: These complementary products are separate from the essential supplements and should be ordered based on the individual needs of each person. All ingredients and current pricing can be found on the web site (www.TheHealthySmoker.net) or provided by a Växa sales representative. 1-877-476-6653.

Ordering Guidelines
Products may be ordered on the web site at:
www.TheHealthySmoker.net.
Products may also be ordered via phone at 1-877-476-6653

Appendix II

Detoxification Formula

Ingredient	Pharmacology	Activators / Used	Carrier Type	Alternate Bio-process	Cautions
Herbal					
Lobelia	Lobelia inflata	Aerial/Roots	phytochemical		
Passion Flower	Passiflora incarnata	Flowers, root, leaves, stem	phytochemical		
Licorice Root	Glycyrrhiza glabra	Root only	phytochemical		Pregnancy, diabetes high blood pressure
Echinacea	Echinacea species	Aerial/Roots	phytochemical		Allergies/ ragweed, sunflower
Ginger Root	Zingiber officinale	Rhizomes	phytochemical		No anticoagulants / Gallstones
Astragalus	Astragalus membranaceus	Root only	phytochemical		Do not take if fever present
Siberian Ginseng	P. Ginseng	Root only	phytochemical		Hyopglycemia, high BP, Asthma
Grape Seed Extract	Oligomeric proanthocyanidins	Flavinoids	phytochemical	Pycnogenol	
Turmeric	Curcuma longa	Rhizomes	phytochemical		
Green Tea	Camillia sinensis	Leaves	phytochemical		
Amino Acids					
L- Glutamine	Glutamic Acid	Acid	N/A	L-Glutamine	
Taurine	Taurine	Acid	N/A	Zinc	
L-Arginine	L-Arginine	Acid	N/A	Open	
Nutriceuticals					
Alpha Lipoic Acid	Same	Acid	Same		
MSM	Methylsulfonylmethane	Sulfur	N/A		
2 Capsules per dose					
60 count bottle					

Special Note: These are the primary ingredients in the detoxification formula. These ingredients may be augmented by a proprietary blend of other herbal or homeopathic ingredients in order to enhance the assimilation and effectiveness of the formula. The complete list of ingredients, strengths and cautions can be found on the website at www.Thehealthysmoker.net, or by asking the sales representatives at Vaxa International. Ingredients are subject to change based on emerging research.

Appendix III
Foods Recommended for Detoxification

Basic Detox Food Guidelines
The diet is low-lactose, low-fat, gluten-free, and usually well tolerated. The primary guidelines are outlined below:

1. Eliminate dairy products such as milk, cheese, and ice cream. (Note: Varying amounts of natural, unsweetened, live-culture yogurt may be tolerated by some individuals.)

2. Avoid meats such as beef, pork, or veal. Chicken, turkey, lamb, and cold-water fish such as salmon, mackerel, and halibut are acceptable if you are not allergic or intolerant of these foods. Select from free-range sources whenever possible.

3. Eliminate gluten. Avoid any food that contains wheat, spelt, kamut, oats, rye, barley, amaranth, or malt. This is the most difficult part of the diet but also the most important. Unfortunately, gluten is contained in many common foods such as bread, crackers, pasta, cereals, and products that contain flour made from these grains. Products made from rice, corn, buckwheat, quinoa, and gluten-free flour, potato, tapioca, and arrowroot may be used as desired, by most individuals.

4. Drink at least two quarts of water, preferably filtered, daily.

5. Avoid all alcohol-containing products, including beer, wine, liquor, and over-the-counter products that contain alcohol. Avoid all caffeine-containing beverages, including coffee, caffeine-containing tea, and soda pop. Coffee substitutes from gluten-containing grains should also be avoided, along with decaffeinated coffee. Read labels carefully, because over-the-counter medications may contain alcohol and/or caffeine.

Sample Detox Meal Plan

Breakfast
1 cup cream of rice, cooked
1 cup soy milk
1 banana

Snack
1 ounce whole blanched almonds

Lunch
2 brown rice cakes with sesame seeds
1 ounce sesame butter (tahini)
1 cup fresh chicken/vegetable/rice soup

Snack
1 Bartlett pear, with skin

Dinner
1 small potato, boiled
1 cup carrots, steamed
6 ounces halibut, broiled
2 cups tossed salad, made from butter lettuce, raw sliced
cucumber, alfalfa sprouts, bell pepper, and sliced tomato. Dressing
of 2 teaspoons olive oil, 1 clove crushed garlic, chopped parsley

Snack
4 ounces pure apple juice or a small cup of unsweetened yogurt.

Total calories: 1350
Carbohydrate: 174 grams, 51% of total
Protein: 91 grams, 27% of total
Fat: 34 grams, 22% of total

Appendix IV

Basic Nutritional Guide

A diet high in nutrients is the key to good health. Use the following table as a guide when deciding which types of food to include in your diet and which ones to avoid in order to maintain good health.

Types of Food	Food to Avoid	Acceptable Foods
Beans	Canned pork and beans, canned beans with salt or preservatives, frozen beans	All beans cooked without animal fat or salt
Beverages	Alcoholic drinks, coffee, cocoa, pasteurized and/ or sweetened juices and fruit drinks, sodas, tea (except herbal tea)	Herbal teas, fresh vegetable and fruit juices, cereal grain beverages (often sold as coffee substitutes) mineral or distilled water
Dairy Products	All soft cheeses, all pasteurized or artificially colored cheese products, ice cream	Raw goat cheese, nonfat cottage cheese, kefir, unsweetened yogurt, goat's milk, raw or skim milk, butter-milk, rice milk, all soy products
Eggs	Fried or pickled	Boiled or poached (limit of 4 weekly)
Fish	All fried fish, all shellfish, salted fish, anchovies, herring, fish canned in oil	All freshwater white fish, salmon, broiled or baked fish, water-packed tuna

Types of Food	Food to Avoid	Acceptable Foods
Fruits	Canned, bottled, or frozen fruits with sweeteners added, oranges	All fresh, frozen, stewed, or dried fruits without sweeteners (except oranges, which are acidic and highly allergenic), unsulfured fruits, home-canned fruits
Grains	All white flour products, white rice, pasta, crackers, cold cereals, instant types of oatmeal, and other hot cereals	All whole grains and products containing whole grains, cereals, breads, muffins, whole-grain crackers, cream of wheat or rye cereal, buckwheat, millet, oats, brown rice, wild rice (limit yeast breads to three servings per week)
Meats	Beef, all forms of pork, hot dogs, luncheon meats, smoked, pickled and processed meats, corned beef, duck, goose, spare ribs, gravies, organ meats	Skinless turkey and chicken, lamb (limit meat to three servings per week)
Nuts	Peanuts, all salted or roasted nuts	All fresh raw nuts (except peanuts)
Oils (fats)	All saturated fats, hydrogenated margarine, refined processed oils, shortenings, hardened oils	All cold-pressed oils, corn, safflower, sesame, olive, flaxseed, soybean, sunflower, canola oils, margarine made from these oils, eggless mayonnaise

168

Types of Food	Food to Avoid	Acceptable Foods
Seasonings	Black or white pepper, salt, hot red peppers, all types of vinegar except pure natural apple cider vinegar	Garlic, onions, cayenne, Spike, all herbs, dried vegetables, apple cider vinegar, tamari, miso, seaweed, dulse
Soups	Canned soups made with salt, preservatives, MSG, or fat stock, all creamed soups	Homemade (salt- and fat-free) bean, lentil, pea, vegetable, barley, brown rice, onion
Sprouts and Seeds	All seeds cooked in oil or salt	All slightly cooked sprouts (except alfalfa, which should be raw and washed thoroughly), wheat-grass, all raw seeds
Sweets	White, brown, or raw cane sugar, corn syrups, chocolate, sugar candy, fructose (except that in fresh whole fruit), all syrups (except pure maple syrup), all sugar substitutes, jams and jellies made with sugar	Barley malt or rice syrup, small amounts of raw honey, pure maple syrup, unsulfered blackstrap molasses
Vegetables	All canned or frozen with salt or additives	All raw, fresh, frozen (no additives), or home canned without salt (undercook vegetables slightly)

Appendix V

Recommended Daily Supplements

Aloe vera – Helps healing and colon cleansing.

Amino acids (as recommended) – Proteins vital to proper cell development.

Bioflavonoids (500 mg/day) – Enhances absorption of vitamin C.

Biotin (300 mg/day) – Aids cell growth and metabolism.

Calcium (1,500 mg/day) – Builds bones and teeth.

Choline (100 mg/day) – Proper transmission of nerve impulses.

Co Q10 (60 mg/day) – Powerful antioxidant and heart protector.

Digestive Enzymes (as recommended) – Aids in digestion and storage of nutrients.

Flaxseed (5,000 mg) – Helps in healing and cell development.

Folic acid (400 mcg/day) – Assists in normal blood formation.

Garlic (as recommended) – Natural antibiotic and lowers blood pressure.

Inositol (100 mg/day) – Reduces cholesterol and promotes hair growth.

Lactobacillus acidophilus – Aids in digestion and absorption of nutrients.

Lecithin (1,200 mg) – Aids in digestion of fats and absorption of vitamins.

Magnesium (1,000 mg/ day) – Helps bone, nerve, and muscle development.

Potassium (90 mg/day) – Helps nervous system and heart rhythm.

Selenium (200 mcg/day) – Antioxidant; protects the immune system.

Silica (as recommended) – Assists assimilation of calcium.

Spirulina (as recommended) – Super nutrient for cleaning and improving the immune system.

Vitamin A (20,000 IU daily) – Prevents age and skin disorders.

Vitamin B1 (50 mg/day) – Enhances circulation and blood formation.

Vitamin B2 (90 mg/day) – Cell growth and particularly eye protection.

Vitamin B3 (100 mg/day) – Proper circulation and healthy skin.

Vitamin B5 (100 mg/day) – Anti-stress help by production of adrenal hormones.

Vitamin B6 (50 mg/day) – Helps develop nervous system and cells generally.

Vitamin B12 (300 mg/day) – Aids cell development and nerve protection.

Vitamin C (3,000 mg/day) – Antioxidant; prevents cancer and heart disease.

Vitamin D (400 IU daily) – Helps calcium build bones and teeth.

Vitamin E (400 IU daily) – Antioxidant; prevents cancer and heart disease.

Zinc (30 mg/day) – Protects prostate and reproductive organs.

Appendix VI

Vitamin A Deficiency Symptoms
- Poor night vision, unable to see well in dim lights.
- Eyes sensitive to glare, sunlight, or bright lights.
- Inability to adjust eyes when entering a dark room.
- Dry eyes.
- Eyelids red, scaly, or dry.
- Eye inflammations, discharge, mattering, eyelids swollen or pus laden.
- Get colds or respiratory infections easily.
- Sinus problems.
- Abscesses in ears, mouth, or salivary glands.
- Brittle hair.
- Dry, rough, or scaly skin.
- Hard "goosebumps" on back of arms that won't go away.
- Acne, pimples, or blackheads.
- Warts.
- Kidney, urinary or bladder infections, burning or itching when urinating.

Vitamin B1 (thiamine) Deficiency Symptoms
- Heart palpitations or gallop rhythm.
- Slow heartbeat or rapid heartbeat.
- Enlarged heart.
- Diastolic blood pressure over 90.
- Forgetfulness, poor memory, short attention span.
- Muscular tenderness, weakness, or wasting.
- Irritability.
- Feel depressed.
- Constipation.
- Loss of appetite or loss of weight.
- Numbness, prickling, or tingling in hands or feet.
- Loss of ankle or knee jerk reflexes.
- Poor coordination.

- Cramping pains in legs.
- Stiffness or swelling in ankles, feet, or legs.
- Tenderness in calf muscle under pressure.

Vitamin B2 (riboflavin) Deficiency Symptoms
- Cracks or sores in corner of mouth.
- Reddish-purple (magenta) -colored tongue.
- Shiny, sore, or swollen tongue.
- Lips red, white, scaly, swollen, or chapped.
- Cataracts.
- Conjunctivitis.
- Sensation of sand on inside of eyelids.
- Eyes sensitive to light or dimming of vision.
- Eyes red, itchy, burning.
- See spots before eyes.
- Red lines in whites of eyes.
- Abnormally greasy or scaly skin around nose.
- Shrinking or "disappearing" upper lip.
- Falling hair, abnormal hair loss.
- Oily hair.

Vitamin B3 (niacin, niacinamide) Deficiency Symptoms
- Diarrhea.
- Indigestion.
- Insomnia.
- Chapping of backs of hands.
- Itchy, red, or inflamed skin, dermatitis.
- Irritability, anxiety, or depression.
- Mental aberrations or schizophrenia.
- Loss of sense of humor.
- Small ulcers or canker sores in mouth.
- Burning sensation in hands or feet.
- Whitish, coated tongue.
- Brilliant red, painful tongue.
- Swollen tongue with red tips and sides.

Vitamin B6 (pyridoxine) Deficiency Symptoms
- Irritability or nervousness.
- Feel confused.
- Can't remember dreams.
- Dizziness.
- Swelling of hands, feet, or ankles (edema).
- Unable to close hands into tight, flat fists.
- Soreness, tenderness, weakness of thumb muscles.
- Greasy scaliness on skin near nose, mouth, eyes.
- Greenish tint to urine.
- Muscular twitching.
- Hyperactivity.
- Poor coordination in walking.
- Female: Nausea of pregnancy.
- Female: Acne worse during periods.

Vitamin B12 (cobalamin) Deficiency Symptoms
- Sore, beefy red tongue.
- Stammer.
- Dizziness.
- Lemon-yellowish tint to skin, pale complexion.
- Numbness, tingling, soreness, or weakness in hands or feet.
- Jerking of limbs.
- Memory loss.
- Anemia.
- Apathy, feel as if you have lost incentive in life.
- Depression, irritability, or moodiness.
- Paranoia, delusions, or hallucinations.
- Loss of appetite.
- Back pains.
- Dimmed vision.
- Confusion, disorientation, or agitation.
- Poor stomach digestion, low stomach acid.
- Female: Menstrual disturbances.

Biotin Deficiency Symptoms
- Skin shiny, dry, and scaly.
- Hair loss.
- Tongue purplish-red (magenta), swollen, and painful.
- Nausea.
- Poor appetite.
- Sleeplessness.
- Muscular pains.
- Mental depression.
- Irregular heartbeat.
- Fingernails a pale color.
- Extreme weakness, exhaustion.

Choline Deficiency Symptoms
- Eczema.
- Bleeding ulcer.
- High blood pressure.
- High cholesterol levels.
- Have difficulty losing weight.

Folic Acid Deficiency Symptoms
- Tongue red, shiny, smooth, and painful.
- Anemia.
- Ulcers in mouth.
- Red, swollen, or bleeding gums.
- Intestinal malabsorption.
- Diarrhea.
- Heart palpitations.
- Lightheadedness, faintness.
- Swelling of ankles.
- Apathy or depression.
- Forgetfulness.
- Loss of appetite, weight loss.
- Graying hair.
- Excess pigmentation of skin.
- Irritable, agitated, brooding, or self-conscious.

PABA (paraaminobenzoic acid) Deficiency Symptoms
* Skin sensitive to sun, photosensitivity.
* Scleroderma.
* White patches on skin, loss of pigment, vitiligo.
* Constipation.
* Depression.
* Irritability.
* Low sex drive.
* Lupus erythematosus.

Pantothenic Acid Deficiency Symptoms
* Pupils in eyes are unusually large, dilated.
* Periods of deep depression.
* Insomnia, sleeplessness.
* Burning sensation of hands or feet.
* Poor coordination.
* Joint pains.
* Muscle cramps.
* Lightheaded or dizzy when getting up from a lying or sitting position.
* Diarrhea or constipation.
* Irritability.
* Headaches.
* Numbness or tingling in hands or feet.
* Rapid heartbeat on exertion.
* Fatigue, tiredness, lack of energy.

Vitamin C Deficiency Symptoms
* Skin bruises easily, "black and blue" marks.
* Hemorrhages or ruptured blood vessels in eye.
* Gums bleed easily, especially when brushing teeth.
* Bluish-red, swollen, and inflamed gums.
* Loose teeth, loss of dental fillings.
* Nosebleeds.
* Cuts, sores, or wounds heal slowly.
* "Fleeting" pains in joints or legs, joint tenderness.

- Catch infections, colds, flu, or viruses easily.
- Listlessness, lack of endurance, tire easily.
- Cuticles tear easily.
- Excessive hair loss.
- Restlessness or irritability.
- Anemia.
- Broken capillaries, hemorrhages, or pink spots on skin.
- Bloating or puffiness in face.
- Fragile bones.

Vitamin D Deficiency Symptoms
- Burning in mouth and throat.
- Joint pains.
- Poor bone development.
- Muscular cramps.
- Rickets (bowlegs, knock-knees).
- Nervousness.
- Abnormal number of dental cavities.
- Insomnia.
- Osteoporosis (demineralized bone).
- Constipation.
- Osteomalacia (softening of bone).
- Nearsightedness, myopia.

Vitamin E Deficiency Symptoms
- Muscular swelling or wasting, muscular dystrophy.
- Brittle and falling hair.
- Hemolytic anemia.
- Female: Menstrual discomfort.
- Male: Low sex drive.

Appendix VII

Supplementary Formula

Supplement Facts: Serving size 3 tablets, Servings per container 40

Amount per serving

Vitamin A
  (100 % Beta Carotene)
Vitamin C
Vitamin D
Vitamin E
Thiamin (Vitamin B-1)
Riboflavin (Vitamin B-2)
Niacin
Vitamin B-6
Folic Acid
Vitamin B-12
Biotin
Pantothenic Acid
Calcium
Iodine
Magnesium
Zinc
Selenium
Copper
Manganese
Chromium
Molybdenum
Potassium
Boron
Choline Bitartrate
Inositol
Spirulina
  Sprouted Barley Juice (dry)
Flaxseed Oil (dry)
Chinese Chiorella (broken cell
  wall)
Bee Pollen
Korean Ginseng (Panax
Ginseng) (root)

PABA
  (Para-Aminobenzoic Acid)
Citrus bioflavinoids
  (Citrus Sinesis) (fruit)
Quercetin (from dimorphandra
  mollis) (fruit)
Rustin Dimorphandra mollis
Hesperidin Complex
  (citrus spp.) (fruit)
Bromelain (Pineapple-
  2000GDU/gm)
Betaine Hydrochloride
Papain (Papaya)
Amylase
Lipase
Protease
Cellulase
Proprietary Lactobacillus Blend
(L. Acidophilus, L. Bifidus,
  L. Blugaricus) (Milk-free: mini-
  mum 1 billion viable Micro-
  organisms per gram at time of
  manufacture)
Oat Bran
Pectin (Apple)
RNA
DNA Wheat Grass Juice (dry)
Carotenoids
Chlorophyll
Vegetable Oil (Borage and
Sunflower) (dry, cold-pressed
  providing Essential Fatty Acids,
  GLA)

Dehydrated Garlic (Allium sativum) (bulb)
Proprietary Herbal Blend
    Echinacea (Echinacea purpurea) (aerial)
    Milk Thistle (Silybum Marianum) (seed)
    Goldenseal (Hydrastis canadensis) (root)
    Ginger Root (Zingiber officinale)
    Ginkgo Biloba (Ginkgo Biloba) (leaf)
    Cayenne Pepper (Capsicum annuum) (fruit)

Special Note: These ingredients constitute the primary nutrients in the sustaining formula which also includes a proprietary blend of additional trace vitamins, minerals and herbs to improve assimilation and effectiveness. These ingredients are subject to ongoing change and upgrades based on emerging research. For more information on all products relative to usage and cautions please go to www.TheHealthySmoker.net.

Chapter References

Chapter I   Can Smokers Really Be Healthy?

Becklake, M., and Lallov, U.: (1990) "The Healthy Smoker: A Phenomenon of Health Selection." American College of Chest Physicians, *Respiration*, 57, B7-144.

Lallov, U.: (2003) "The Cough Reflex and the Healthy Smoker." American College of Chest Physicians, *Chest*,123:660-662.

Vaccarella, Joseph: (1996) *Introducing Healthy Influence on a Cigarette Smoker.* Author.

Chapter II   The Strength of Smoking's Addiction

Benowitz N. L.: (1988) "Pharmacologic Aspects of Cigarette Smoking and Nicotine Addiction." *New England Journal of Medicine*, 319:1318-30.

Centers for Disease Control and Prevention, National Center for Chronic Disease Prevention and Health Promotion: (2001) "Tobacco Information and Prevention Source." Online at: http://www.cdc.gov/tobacco/issue.htm.

"Cigarette Maker Concedes Smoking Can Cause Cancer/Admits Tobacco is Addictive." *New York Times*, A1, March 21, 1997.

Department of Health and Human Services, Public Health Services: "Why People Smoke Cigarettes." Washington, DC: U.S. Government Printing Office, revised 1984 (No. 83-50195).

Giovino, G. A., Henningfield, J. E., Tomar, S. L., Escobedo, L. G., and Slade, J.: (1995) "Epidemiology of Tobacco Use and Dependence." *Epidemiology Review,* 17:282-93.

"How We Get Addicted." *Time*, May 5, 1997.

Hughes, J. R.: (1994) "Nicotine Withdrawal, Dependence, and Abuse," in *DSM-IV Sourcebook, vol. 1.* Edited by T. A. Widiger, A. J. Frances, H. A. Pincus, M. B. First, R. Ross, and W. Davis. Washington, DC: American Psychiatric Association, 109-116.

Hughes, J. R.: (1993) "Smoking as a Drug Dependence: A Reply to Robinson and Pritchard." *Psychopharmacology* (Berl), 113:282-283.

Kozlowski, L., Wilkinson, D., Skinner, D., Kent, C., Franklin, T., and Pope, M.: (1989) "Comparing Tobacco Cigarette Dependence With Other Drug Dependence." *Journal of the American Medical Association,* 261:898-901.

"Many Smokers Who Can't Quit Are Mentally Ill." *New York Times,* Aug. 27, 1997.

Warburton, D. M.: "The Function of Smoking." *Advances in Behavioral Biology,* 31: 51-61.

Martin, W. R., Vanboon, G. R., Swamoto, E. T., and Davis, L., eds.: (1987) *Tobacco Smoking and Nicotine: A Neurobiological Approach.* New York: Plenum Press.

Chapter III   Smoking's Impact on Your Body

"Cigarettes: What the Warning Label Doesn't Tell You." *American Council of Science and Health.* (1995).

Balin, A. K., and Kligman, A. M.: (1989) *Aging and the Skin.* New York: Raven Press.

Colditz, G. A., Bonita, R., Stampfer, M. J., et al.: (1988) "Cigarette Smoking and Risk of Stroke in Middle-Aged Women." *New England Journal of Medicine,* 318:937-41.

Council on Scientific Affairs: (1990) "The Worldwide Smoking Epidemic: Tobacco Trade, Use and Control." *Journal of the American Medical Association,* 263:3312-18.

Department of Health and Human Services, Public Health Services. (1988) "The Health Consequences of Smoking: Nicotine Addiction: A Report of the Surgeon General." Washington DC: U.S. Government Printing Office (CDC 88-8406).

Department of Health and Human Services: "The Health Consequences of Smoking: 25 Years of Progress." U.S. Government Printing Office (89-8411).

Kadunce, D. P., Burr, R., Gress, R., Kanner, R., Lyon, J. L., and Zone, J. J.: (1991) "Cigarette Smoking: Risk Factor for Premature Facial Wrinkling." *Annals of Internal Medicine,* 114: 840-44.

Facelmann, K. A.: (1991) "Two New Wrinkles for Cigarette Smokers." *Science News,* May 18, 1991.

Fielding, J., and Phenow, K. J.: (1988) "Health Effects of Involuntary Smoking." *New England Journal of Medicine,* 319:1452-60.

Frye, R. E., Schwartz, B. S., and Doty, R. L.: (1990) "Dose-related Effects of Cigarette Smoking on Olfactory Function." *Journal of the American Medical Association,* 263 (9):1233-36.

"How Hazardous is Smoking?" (1996) Mayo Clinic Family Health/Mayo Foundation for Medical Education and Research.

Dollery, C., and Brennan, P. J.: (1988) "The Medical Research Council Hypertension Trial: The Smoking Patient." *American Heart Journal,* 115: 276-81.

"Decreased Clinical Efficacy of Propoxyphene in Cigarette Smokers." (1973) *Clinical Pharmacology and Therapeutics,* 14: 259-63.

Eiserich, J. P., van der Vliet, A., Handelman, G. J., et al.: (1995) "Dietary Antioxidants and Cigarette Smoke-induced Bimolecular Damage: A Complex Interaction." *American Journal of Clinical Nutrition,* 62 (suppl.):1490S-1500S.

Frye, R. E., Schwartz, B. S., and Doty, R. L.: (1990) "Dose-related Effects of Cigarette Smoking on Olfactory Function." *Journal of the American Medical Association,* 263 (9):1233-36.

Handelman, G. J., Packet, L., and Cross, C. E.: (1996) "Destruction of Tocopherols, Carotenoids and Retinal in Human Plasma by Cigarette Smoke." *American Journal of Clinical Nutrition,* 63:559-565.

Lin, H. J.: (1996) "Smokers and Breast Cancer. Chemical Individuality and Cancer Predisposition." *Journal of the American Medical Association,* 276:1511-12.

Office of Health and Environmental Assessment: (1992) "Respiratory Health Effects of Passive Smoking: Lung Cancer and Other Disorders." Washington, DC: U.S. Government Printing Office.

Omenn, G. S., Goodman, G. E., Thornquist, M.D., Balmes, J., Cullen, M. R., Glass, A., Keogh J. P., Meyskens, Jr., F. L., Valanis, B., Williams, Jr., J. H., et al.: (1996) "Risk Factors Lung Cancer and for Intervention Effects in CARET, the Beta-Carotene and Retinol Efficacy Trial." *Journal of the National Cancer Institute,* 88 (21):1550-59.

Swanson, J. A., Lee, J. W., Hopp, J. W., and Berk, L. S.: (1997) "The Impact of Caffeine Use On Tobacco Cessation and Withdrawal." *Addictive Behaviors,* 1:55-68.

Chapter IV   Testing the Health of Smokers

King, M., Barrager, E., Bland, J., and Medcalf, D.: *Correlation of the Metabolic Screening Questionnaire (MSQ) as an Instrument for Evaluating Health Outcomes in Comparison to the Medical Outcome Survey (MOS).* In press.

Wilson, I, and Cleary, P.: (1995) "Linking Clinical Variables with Health-Related Quality of Life - A Conceptual Model of Patient Outcomes." *Journal of the American Medical Association,* 273:59-65.

Chapter V   Detoxification Before Anything Else

Baker, M. D., and MacDonald, S.: (1997) *Detoxification and Healing.* New Canaan, CT: Keats Publishing.

Bland, J., Barranger, E., Reedy, R. G., and Blank, K.: (1995) "A Medical Food Supplemented Detoxification Program in the Management of Chronic Health Problems." *Alternative Therapies in Health and Medicine,* 1:62-71.

Brown, L., Rowe, A., Ryle, P., et al.: (1983) "Efficacy of Vitamin Supplementation in Chronic Alcoholics Undergoing Detoxification." *Alcohol,* 18:157-166.

Church, D. F., and Pryor, W. A.: (1985) "Free Radical Chemistry of Cigarette Smoke and Its Toxicological Implications." *Environmental Health Perspectives,* 64:111-26.

Davis, R.: (1998) "Exposure to Environmental Tobacco Smoke." *The Journal of the American Medical Association,* 280 (22).

Guengerich, F. P.: (1984) "Effects of Nutritive Factors on Metabolic Processes Involving Bioactivation and Detoxification of Chemicals." *Annual Review of Nutrition,* 4:207-231.

Halliwell, F., and Getteridge, J. M. C., eds.: (1998) *Free Radicals in Biology and Medicine,* 3rd ed. Oxford, England: Clarendon Press.

Odeleye, O., Eskelson, C., and Watson, R.: (1993) "Alcohol Ingestion and Lipoperoxidation: Role of Glutathione in Antioxidant Defense and Detoxification." *Journal of Optimum Nutrition,* 2:173-189.

Page, L.: (2002) *Detoxification*. Carmel Valley, CA: Traditional Wisdom.

Parpalei, P. A., et al.: (1991) "The Use of Sauna for Disease Prevention in the Workers of Enterprises with Chemical and Physical Occupational Hazards." *Vrach. Delo.,* 5: 93-95.

Schnare, D. W., et al.: (1982) "Evaluation of a Detoxification Regimen for Fat Stored Xenobiotics." *Medical Hypotheses,* 9:265-82.

Spitz, D. R., Sullivan, S. J., Malcolm, R. R., and Roberts, R. J.: (1991) "Glutathione Dependent Metabolism and Detoxification of 4-Hydroxy-2-Nonenal." *Free Radical Biology & Medical,* 11:415-423.

Stockwell, T., Bolt, L., and Milner, I., et al.: (1990) "Home Detoxification for Problem Drinkers: Acceptability to Clients, Relatives, General Practitioners, and Outcome After 60 Days." *British Journal on Addiction,* 85:61-70.

Chapter VI   The Digestive System

Gottschall, E.: (1986) *Food and the Gut Reaction.* Kirkton, Ontario, Canada: The Kirkton Press.

Gottschall, E.: (1994) *Breaking the Vicious Cycle: Intestinal Health Through Diet.* Kirkton, Ontario, Canada: The Kirkton Press.

Jensen, B.: (1999) *Dr. Jensen's Guide to Better Bowel Care.* New York: Avery.

Kikendall, J. W., Evaul, J., and Johnson, L. F.: (1984) "Effects of Cigarette Smoking on Gastrointestinal Physiology and Non-Neoplastic Digestive Tissue." *Journal of Clinical Gastro-enterology,* 6:65-79.

Treneu, N.: (1998) *Probiotics.* Garden City Park, NY: Avery.

Chapter VII   Nutritional Guidelines for Smokers

Balch, J. F., and Balch, P. A.: (1997) *Prescription for Nutritional Healing.* Garden City Park, NY: Avery.

Berlan, M., et al.: (1995) "Lipid Mobilization, Physiopathological and Pharmacological Aspects." *Annual Endocrinology,* 56:97-100.

Bland, J. S.: (1999) *Genetic Nutritioneering.* Los Angeles: Keats Publishing.

Bland, J., and Benum, S.: (1996) *The 20-day Rejuvenation Diet Program.* New Canaan, CT: Keats Publishing.

Block, G., Patterson, B., and Sufar, A.: (1992) "Fruit, Vegetables, and Cancer Prevention: A Review of the Epidemiological Evidence." *Journal of Nutrition and Cancer,* 18:1-29.

Carr, A. C., and Frie, B.: (1999) "Toward a New Recommended Dietary Allowance for Vitamin C Based on Antioxidant and Health Effects in Humans." *American Journal of Clinical Nutrition,* 69:1086-107.

Church, M.: (2004) *Adrenaline Junkies & Serotonin Seekers.* Berkeley, CA: Ulysses Press.

Dempsey, D. T., Mullen, J. L., and Buzby, G. P., et al.: (1988) "The Link Between Nutritional Status and Clinical Outcome: Can Nutritional Intervention Modify It?" *American Journal of Clinical Nutrition,* 47:352-356.

Holford, P.: (1999) *The Optimum Nutrition Bible.* Freedom, CA: The Crossing Press.

Jarvinen, R., Seppanen, R., Hellovaara, M., Teppo, L., Pukkala, E., and Aromaa, A.: (1997) "Dietary Flavonoids and the Risk of Lung Cancer and Other Malignant Neoplasms." *American Journal of Epidemiology,* 146 (3):223-30.

Kolonel, L. N., Marchand, L., Hankin, J. H., Bach, F., Wilkins, L., Stacewicz, M., Bowen, P., Beecher, L. S., Lauden, F., Baques, P., Daniel, R., Serunatu, L., and Henderson, B.: (1991) "Relation of Nutrient Intakes and Smoking in Relation to Cancer Incidence in Cook Islanders." *Proceedings of the American Association for Cancer Research,* 37:1369-71.

Lockwood, K., Moesgaard, S., Hanioka, T., and Folkers, K.: (1994) "Apparent Partial Remission of Breast Cancer in "High Risk" Patients Supplemented with Nutritional Antioxidants, Essential Fatty Acids and Coenzyme Q10." *Molecular Aspects of Medicine,* 15 (suppl.):S231-40.

Madhavi, D. L., Deshpande, S. S., and Salunkhe, D. K., eds.: (1996) *Food Antioxidants: Technological, Toxicological and Health Perspectives.* New York: Marcel Dekker.

Ohigashi, H., Osawa, T., Terao, J., Watanabe, S., and Yoshikawa, T., eds.: (1997) *Food Factors for Chemistry and Cancer Prevention.* Tokyo: Springer-Verlag.

Packer, L., ed.: (1995) "Biothiols: Monothiols and Dithiols, Protein Tthiols and Thiyl Radicals." *Methods in Enzymology, v*ol. 251. San Diego: Academic Press.

Pappas, A., ed.: (1998) *Antioxidant Status, Diet, Nutrition, and Health.* Boca Raton, FL: CRC Press.

Pryor, K.: (1999) "Serrapeptase: Insect-Derived Enzyme Fights Inflammation." *Vitamin Research Products,* December: 1-15.

Pryor, W. A.: (1991) "The Antioxidant Nutrients and Disease Prevention – What Do We Know and What Do We Need to Find Out?" *American Journal of Clinical Nutrition,* 53 (suppl. 1):391-93.

Rajagopalan, K. V.: (1988) "Molybdenum: An Essential Trace Element in Human Nutrition." *Annual Review of Nutrition,* 8:401-427.

Regnstrom, J., Nilsson, J., Moldeus, P., Strom, K., Bavenholm, P., Tornvall, P., and Hamsten, A.: (1996) "Inverse Relation Between the Concentration of Low-Density-Lipoprotein Vitamin E and Severity of Coronary Artery Disease." *American Journal of Clinical Nutrition,* 63 (3):377-85.

Rice-Evans, C., and Packer, L., eds.: (1997) "Flavonoids in Health and Disease." In Vol. 7 of *Antioxidants in Health and Disease,* edited by L. Packer and J. Fuchs. New York: Marcel Dekker.

Willett, W.: *Nutritional Epidemiology.* 2nd ed. New York: Oxford University Press.

Willett, W., et al.: (1995) "Mediterranean Diet Pyramid: A Cultural Model for Healthy Eating." *American Journal of Clinical Nutrition,* 61 (suppl): 51402-6.

Chapter VIII   The Importance of Supplementation

The Alpha-Tocopherol, Beta Carotene Cancer Prevention Study Group: (1994) "The Effect of Vitamin E and Beta Carotene on the Incidence of Lung Cancer and Other Cancers in Male Smokers." *New England Journal of Medicine,* 330 (15):1029-35.

Anand, C. L.: (1971) "Effect of Avena Sativa on Cigarette Smoking." *Nature,* 233:496.

Balch, J., and Balch, A.: (1997) *Prescription for Nutritional Healing Antioxidants.* Avery. Garden City, New York.

Bendich, A., and Langseth, L.: (1995) "The Health Effects of Vitamin C Supplementation: A Review." *Journal of the American College of Nutrition,* 14:124-36.

Blomhoff, R., ed.: (1994) "Vitamin A in Health and Disease." In Vol. 1 of *Antioxidants in Health and Disease,* edited by L. Packer and J. Fuchs. New York: Marcel Dekker.

Brown, A. J.: (1996) "Acute Effects of Smoking Cessation on Antioxidant Status." *Experimental Journal of Nutritional Biochemistry,* 7:29-39.

Burk, R. F., ed.: (1994) *Selenium in Biology and Human Health.* New York: Springer-Verlag.

Cadenas, E., and Packer, L., eds.: (1996) "Handbook of Antioxidants." In Vol. 3 of *Antioxidants in Health and Disease,* edited by L. Packer and J. Fuchs. New York: Marcel Dekker.

Chandra, R.: (1997) "Nutrition and the Immune System: An Introduction." *American Journal of Clinical Nutrition,* (66) 478-484.

Coursin, D. B., & Cihla, H. P.: (1996). "Pulmonary Effects of Short-Term Selenium Deficiency." *Thorax,* 51(5): 479-83.

Davison, G. C., and Rosen, R. C.: (1972) "Lobeline and Reduction of Cigarette Smoking." *Psychology Report,* 31:443-456.

Editors of *Prevention Magazine*: (1996) *Healing with Vitamins.* Emmaus, PA: Rodale Press.

Fuchs, J., Packer, L., and Zimmer, G., eds.: (1997) "Lipoic Acid in Health and Disease." In Vol. 6 of *Antioxidants in Health and Disease,* edited by L. Packer and J. Fuchs. New York: Marcel Dekker.

Fuchs, J. and Packer, L., eds.: (1991) *Vitamin C in Health and Disease,* vol. 5. New York: Marcel Dekker.

Garland, M., Stampfer, M. J., Willett, W. C., and Hunter, D. J.: (1994) "The Epidemiology of Selenium and Human Cancer." In *Natural Antioxidants in Human Health and Disease,* edited by B. Frei. New York: Academic Press.

Grandjean, E. M., et al.: (2000). "Efficacy of Oral Long Term N-Acetylcysteine in Chronic Bronchiopulmonary Disease: A Meta-Analysis of Published Double-blind, Placebo-controlled Clinical Trials." *Clinical Therapeutics,* 22(2):209-21.

Haramaki, N., Packer, L., Droy-Lefaix, M. T., and Christen, T.: (1996) *Antioxidant Actions and Health Implications of Ginkgo Biloba Extract.* In *Handbook of Antioxidants,* edited by E. Cadenas and L. Packer. New York: Marcel Dekker.

Hosseini, S., et al. (2001). "Pycnogenol in the Management of Asthma." *Journal of Medicinal Food,* 4(4):201-9.

Johnston, C. S., Meyer, C. G., and Srilakshmi, J. C.: (1993) "Vitamin C Elevates Red Blood Cell Glutathione in Healthy Adults." *American Journal of Clinical Nutrition,* 58 (1):103-05.

Keli, S. O., Hertog, M. G., Feskens, E. J., and Kromhout, D.: (1996) "Dietary Flavonoids, Antioxidant Vitamins, and Incidence of Stroke: The Zutphen Study." *Archives of Internal Medicine,* 156 (6): 637-42.

Knekt, P., Marniemi, J., Teppo, L., Heliovaara, M., and Aromaa, A.: (1998) "Is Low Selenium a Risk Factor of Lung Cancer?" *American Journal of Epidemiology,* 148 (10).

Krinsky, N. I., and Sies, H., eds.: (1995) "Antioxidant Vitamins and Beta Carotene in Disease Prevention." *American Journal of Clinical Nutrition,* 62(6)Suppl:1299S-1540S.

Mayne, S. T.: (1996) "Beta-carotene, Carotenoids and Disease Prevention in Humans." *The Federation of American Societies for Experimental Biology (FASEB) Journal,* 10:690-701.

Multicenter Study Group. (1980). "Long Term Oral Acetylcysteine in Chronic Bronchitis: A Double-blind Controlled Study." *European Journal of Respiratory Disease,* 61(Suppl 111): 93-108.

Packer, L., and Fuchs, J., eds.: (1991) *Vitamin C in Health and Disease,* vol. 5. New York: Marcel Dekker.

Packer, L., and Colman, C.: (1999) *The Antioxidant Miracle.* New York: John Wiley & Sons.

Pauling L.: (1968) "Orthomolecular Psychiatry." *Science,* 160:265.

Sinatra, S. T. (1998) *The Coenzyme Q10 Phenomenon.* New Canaan, CT: Keats Publishing.

Sreejayan, R.: (1997) "Nitric Oxide Scavenging by Curcuminoids." *Journal of Pharmaceutical Pharmacology,* 49:105-107.

Wu, D., Meydani, S. N., Sastre, J., Hayek, M., and Meydani, M.: (1994) "In Vitro Glutathione Supplementation Enhances Interleukin-2 Production and Mitogenic Response of Peripheral Blood Mononuclear Cells from Young and Old Subjects." *Journal of Nutrition,* 124 (5): 655-63.

Chapter IX   The Importance of Exercise

ACSM: (1988) "Position Stand on the Recommended Quantity and Quality of Exercise for Developing and Maintaining Cardiorespiratory and Muscular Fitness and Flexibility in Healthy Adults." *Medicine and Science in Sports and Exercise,* 30:975-991.

Allen, J., Schnyer, R., and Hitt, S.: (1998) "The Efficacy of Acupuncture in the Treatment of Major Depression in Women." *Psychology as Science,* 9:397-401.

American College of Sports Medicine: (1986) *Guidelines for Exercise, Testing and Prescription.* Philadelphia: Lea & Febiger.

Blair, S., Kohl, H., Paffenbarger, R., et al.: (1989) "Physical Fitness and All-cause Mortality." *Journal of the American Medical Association,* 262:2395-2401.

Centers for Disease Control and Prevention: (1999) "Public Health Focus: Effectiveness of Smoking-control Strategies – United States." *Morbidity & Mortality Weekly Report,* 41(35):645-647,653.

Dunlap, J., and Barry, H.: (1999) "Overcoming Exercise Barriers in Older Adults." *Physician Sports Medicine,* 27:69-75.

Rippe, J., Ward, A., Porcuri, H., and Freedson, P. S.: (1988) "Walking for Health and Fitness." *Journal of the American Medical Association,* 259:2720-24.

Sen, C., Packer, L., and Hanninen, O., eds.: (1994) *Exercise and Oxygen Toxicity.* Amsterdam: Elsevier.

U.S. Department of Health and Human Services: (1996) *Physical Activity and Health: A Report of the Surgeon General.* Atlanta: Centers for Disease Control and Prevention.

U.S. Preventative Services Task Force: (1996) *Guide to Clinical Preventative Services,* 2nd ed. Baltimore: Williams and Wilkins.

Chapter X   Natural Therapies for Smokers

Bensen, H.: (1975) *The Relaxation Response.* New York: Avon Books.

Davis, P.: (1988) *Aromatherapy, An A-Z.* Saffron Walden, England: C. W. Daniels.

Diamond, J. L., Cowden, W. L., and Goldberg, B.: (1997) *An Alternative Medicine Definitive Guide to Cancer.* Tiburon, CA: Future Medicine Publishing.

Editors of Prevention Magazine Health Books: (1995) *Fighting Disease.* Emmaus, PA: Rodale Press.

Haus, F., and Sherber, S.: (1990) *The Chronic Bronchitis and Emphysema Handbook.* New York: John Wiley & Sons.

Hawkeye, S.: (1997) *Herbalism.* London, England: Lorenz Books.

Hoffman, D.: (2000) *Easy Breathing.* Pownal, VT: Storey Books.

Hoffman, E., and Hoffman, C.: (1998) *Recovery From Smoking.* Center City, MN: Hazeldon.

Hudson, J.: (1996) *Instant Meditation for Stress Relief.* London, England: Lorenz Books.

Jendricks, G.: (1995) *Conscious Breathing.* New York: Bantam.

Larson, J. M.: (1999) *Depression Free Naturally.* New York: Random House.

Maccaro, J.: (2003) *Natural Health Remedies.* Lake Mary, FL: Silvam.

Marks, C.: (2002) *Homeopathy: A Step By Step Guide.* London: Elements Books.

McVicker, M.: (1997) *Sauna Detoxification Therapy.* Jefferson, NC: McFarland and Co.

Meyer, R.: (1992) *Practical Clinical Hypnosis: Techniques and Applications.* New York: Lexington Books, Macmillan.

Ornish, D.: (1990) *Program for Reversing Heart Disease.* New York: Ballantine Books.

Pittler, M., and Ernst, E.: (2000) "Efficacy of Kava Extract for Treating Anxiety: Systematic Review and Meta-Analysis."

Journal of Clinical Psychopharmacology, 20:84-89.

Pryor, K.: (1999). "Serrapeptase: Insect-Derived Enzyme Fights Inflammation." *Vitamin Research Products,* December: 1-15.

Rakel, D.: (2003) *Integrative Medicine.* New York: Saunders.

Ramirez, L., Mulrow, G., et al.: (1996) "St. John's Wort for Depression — An Overview and Meta-Analysis of Randomized Clinical Trials." *British Medical Journal,* 313:253-258.

Rea, W., Pan,Y., Johnson, A., et al.: (1996) "Reduction of Chemical Sensitivity by Means of Heat Deprivation, Physical Therapy, and Nutritional Supplementation in a Controlled Environment." *Journal of Nutrition and Environmental Medicine,* 6: 141-148.

Reilly, D.: (1997) *The Foundation of Homeopathy,* 15th ed. Glasgow: Acthom Ltd.

Rowlands, B.: (1999) *Alternative Answers to Asthma &Allergies.* London: Marshal Editions Development.

Shwartz, M., Suitz, R., and Brannigan, P.: (1998) "The Value of Acupuncture Detoxification Programs in a Substance Abuse Treatment System." *Journal of Substance Abuse Treatment,* 17:305-312.

Smyth, J., Stone, A., Hurcivitz, A., and Kaell, A.: (1999) "Effects of Writing About Stressful Experiences on Symptom Reduction in Patients with Asthma and Rheumatoid Arthritis." *Journal of the American Medical Association,* 281:1304-1309.

Stangler, M.: (2001) *The Natural Physician's Healing Therapies.* Stanford, CT: Prentice Hall Press.

Wanning, E.: (1994) *Meditations for Surviving Without Cigarettes.* New York: Avon Books.

Wellness Councils of America: (2001) *Quitting Smoking.* Omaha, NE.

Chapter XI   Managing Your Habit

"Practice Guideline for the Treatment of Patients With Nicotine Dependence." (1996) *American Psychiatric Association,* 23-28.

Gray, J.: (2003) *The Mars & Venus Diet and Exercise Solution.* New York: St. Martins Press.

Hughes, J., and Hatsukamis, D.: (1992) "The Nicotine Withdrawal Syndrome: A Brief Review and Update." *International Journal of Smoking Cessation,* 1:21-26.

Perkins, K.: (1994) "Issues in the Prevention of Weight Gain After Smoking Cessation." *Annals of Behavioral Medicine,* 16:46-52.

Chase Cancer Center and funded by the Pennsylvania Department of Health: (1987) "Quitting Times: A Magazine for Women Who Smoke." *National Institutes of Health,* 89-1647.

Schwartz, G.: (1975) "Biofeedback, Self-Regulation, and Patterning of Physiological Processes." *American Science,* 63:314-24.

Tobacco Use and Dependence Clinical Practice Guideline Update Panel and Staff.: (2000) "A Clinical Practice Guideline for Treating Tobacco Use and Dependence." *Journal of the American Medical Association,* (283) 24.

Westermeyer, R.: *Smoking Reduction Tips.* La Jolla, CA:

Chapter XII   The Psychology of Quitting

Carr, A.: (2004) *The Easy Way to Stop Smoking.* New York: Sterling.

Convey, L. S., Glassman, A. H., and Stetner, F.: (1997) "Major Depression Following Smoking Cessation." *American Journal of Psychiatry,* 154, 2:263-265.

Ferguson, T.: (1989) *The No-Nag, No Guilt, Do-It-Your-Own-Way Guide to Quitting Smoking.* New York: Ballantine Books.

U.S. Department of Health and Human Services: (1990) *Health Benefits of Smoking Cessation: A Report of the U.S. Surgeon General.* Washington, DC, U.S. Government Printing Office.

Department of Health and Human Services: *The Health Consequences of Smoking: 25 Years of Progress.* 89-8411. Washington, DC: U.S. Government Printing Office.

Hoffman, E., Blackburn, C., and Cullari, S.: (1997) "Five Year Follow Up Study of Brief Residential Nicotine Treatment." *Journal of Addictive Diseases,* 16 (4):18A. (Other publications of this research are in progress).

Klesges, R., Ward, K., and DeBon, M.: (1996) "Smoking Cessation: A Successful Behavioral/Pharmacologic Interface." *Clinical Psychology Review,* 16:479-496.

Chapter XIII Cessation – Much Easier Now

How to Stop Smoking. (1996) Mayo Clinic Family Health/Mayo Foundation for Medical Education and Research.

American College of Physicians, Health and Policy Committee: (1986) "Methods for Stopping Cigarette Smoking." *Annual Internal Medicine,* 105:281-291.

"Patches Aid Smoking Cessation in General Practice." *Journal Watch,* June 25, 1993.

Rustin, T.: (1991) *Quit and Stay Quit.* Center City, MN.

Smoking Cessation: A Guide for Primary Care Physicians. U.S. Dept of Health and Human Services; AHCPR publication No. 96-0693.

The Health Benefits of Smoking Cessation. (1990) Centers for Disease Control. U.S. Dept of Health and Human Services. CDC 90-8416.

"Transdermal Nicotine for Smoking Cessation." *Journal Watch,* May 10, 1991.

"Which Nicotine Patch Users Will Stop Smoking?" *Journal Watch*, October 28, 1996.